HOW TO KEEP YOUR
BAD HABITS

AND STILL AVOID FLAME-OUT

(The **Nutritional** Connection)

HOW TO KEEP YOUR
BAD HABITS

AND STILL AVOID FLAME-OUT

(The **Nutritional** Connection)

by
David A. Keiper

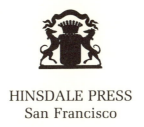

HINSDALE PRESS
San Francisco

NOTE

This book is not intended to replace medical diagnosis and treatment. For possible serious health problems, readers must consult a physician.

The author is a research scientist, not an M. D. He is presenting research findings, interpreting data, and offering ideas (some of which are speculative). A personal physician is best situated to recognize subtle differences between individuals, and determine application in each case.

Copyright © 1986 by David A. Keiper

Printed in the United States of America

1 2 3 4 5 6 7 8 9 10

Library of Congress Cataloging in Publication Data

Keiper, David A.
   How to keep your bad habits and still avoid flame-out (the nutritional connection)

   Bibliography: p.
   Includes Index.
   1. Coronary heart disease--Nutritional aspects.
2. Coronary heart disease--Diet therapy. 3. Vitamins in human nutrition. 4. Minerals in human nutrition.
I. Title.
RC685.C6K35 1986   616.1'23   85-17605
ISBN 0-931375-16-9 (alk. paper)
ISBN 0-931375-17-7 (pbk. : alk. paper)

Cover design by George L. Stewart

ACKNOWLEDGEMENTS. I owe much to all the researchers whose work I've used. Some of their names will be found among the references. Any errors in interpreting their work are strictly my own.

Thanks to my wife, Mary, for her patience and her help, and to the friends who've read and commented upon the manuscript. The ones who have contributed the most are: Robert E. Beck, Knud D. Dyby, Ralph A. Hohmann, Lynn C. Motai, Terry Norbury, Edmond J. Scola, and Richmond W. Smith, Jr, M. D.

SUMMARY

The book addresses the serious question of why men are dying more than seven years younger than women, on average. The major reason lies in the greater vulnerability of the male to coronary heart disease in industrialized countries. Behind it are certain nutritional factors (other than fat and cholesterol) that have undergone drastic changes over the past century. The data appear to hold worldwide, and thus the factors the author has identified offer a resolution of the diet-heart controversies. These factors appear far more important than so-called bad habits—smoking, drinking, stress, lack of exercise, etc. The book covers the needed dietary changes for promoting heart health, the interactions of the bad habits with nutritional factors, and the nutritional therapies that slow down aging and are useful in treating many different ailments.

The book is written for a general audience, but includes technical notes and references for health professionals.

Contents

INTRODUCTION   1

1. TOO MANY EXPERTS   3
2. THE BIGGEST RISKS   7
3. HELPING MEN LIVE LONGER   11
4. STAYING OUT OF TROUBLE   16
5. MAN MUDDLES THROUGH   20
6. THE CHEMISTRY OF LIFE   27
7. DIETARY DRIFT   37
8. MORE ABOUT MINERALS   46
9. THE SACRED COW   53
10. CONTROLLING CHOLESTEROL   59
11. FEAR OF FATS   63
12. 'BAD HABIT' SCOREBOARD   67
13. KEEPING YOUR HEAD STRAIGHT   81
14. SEX AND NUTRITION   87
15. ASSORTED HAZARDS   98
16. ENJOYMENT OF FOOD   104
17. INDIVIDUALIZED NUTRITIONAL THERAPY   114
18. PROPER USE OF SUPPLEMENTS   119
19. BEATING THE ODDS   140

Appendix I. TOWARD A UNIFIED HYPOTHESIS   145
OF CORONARY HEART DISEASE
Appendix II. ASSESSING YOUR   153
NUTRITIONAL STATE
REFERENCE NOTES   162
INDEX   178

To my father and my uncle,
who left this world too soon,
victims of heart disease.

To my young son, who will
hopefully never have to
worry about such matters.

Introduction

Have you ever wondered how some people seem to get away with all kinds of bad habits? No doubt you've felt envy at times. But are they really getting away with high living, or will there be a later reckoning? They could be headed for serious health problems as they age——or an early death. A few may get off scot-free——those who have inherited an iron constitution. But for us ordinary mortals, is there a way that we can extend our usual limits? There certainly is. And someone with an iron constitution is apt to come close to becoming Superman.

Now, when I say extending our limits, I mean something other than being able to drink others under the table without ill effects. I mean that you can achieve optimum health——a state in which your body is best able to withstand all the insults thrown at it, whether they come from bad habits, stress, or exposure to environmental pollutants. This book will tell you how to achieve optimum health——enabling you to live longer and, more importantly, helping you to avoid various infirmities that tend to come with aging.

In the case of men, modern medicine has failed them. The life expectancy of women has been extended far more than that of men in the past half century. American men die more than seven years younger than women, on average. Yet back in 1920, there was only a one year difference. Typically, male "bad habits" are blamed for much of the sizable difference in life expectancy. As you read on, you'll find that bad habits are only a small part of the problem.

1

Now, don't get me wrong: I am not recommending bad habits.   Men or women who have too many of them may suffer a deterioration in health or an early death.   It is impossible to say what is "too many" for any individual.   In some cases we get warning signs of our limits and can slow down a bit.   But the problem is, many times there are no warning signs—especially true of sudden cardiac death, the biggest male killer in the middle years.

The one habit you can't get away with is the modern civilized diet.   It is much worse than the worst of the usual "bad habits."   Frankly, I'm almost afraid to use the word "diet," since that word calls up images of people giving up all sorts of foods they enjoy.   Most likely, you'll be pleasantly surprised with the modest dietary changes that we need.   Many nutritionists mistakenly lay a bum rap on foods containing fat and cholesterol.   (More on that later.)   Also, men have somewhat different nutritional needs than women, but few nutritionists seem to appreciate the full extent of the differences.

Complicating the story are the vast differences between individuals.   This is especially true of our nutritional needs.   Thus you must ultimately become the expert on your own body and its needs.   However, for the present, let me guide you in the search for your own optimum nutrition.   Along the way, I will help you understand the workings of your body and your mind, so that you may develop good independent judgment on health and nutrition.

Armed with this knowledge, you will be able to discover the foods on which you can thrive.   You will learn to use vitamin and mineral supplements wisely.   With this balanced account of so-called bad habits, you will be able to assess your own risks.   The book can also help you dump any habits which you decide are messing up your life.   You'll be able to liberate yourself from worrying about most of the scare stuff that appears in the media.

Although the book focuses on male health problems, women will wish to read it, for much applies to them.   The book is also for women who want to help the men in their lives stay healthy and alive.

CHAPTER 1

Too Many Experts

On all sides, people have been telling you that you have to give up smoking, drinking, type "A" behavior, trim your weight down, get more exercise, or quit eating certain foods that have fat, cholesterol, salt, or sugar in them. Others tell you to watch out for the additives, preservatives, or pesticides in your food. Still other experts warn you about the air you breathe and the water you drink.

How in the world could you ever follow all those warnings? No doubt, you'd like to shut all the experts out of your mind. Should you consider giving up some of your pleasures? Maybe you feel guilty as you sneak some forbidden item. At any time now you expect some expert to come out with: "Warning! Living may be hazardous to your health."

The implied threat, if you ignore their warnings, is that you may suffer **flame-out.** I've borrowed this apt term from jet-engine technology. Flame-out is the sudden loss of power of a jet aircraft on take-off or in flight. The result is a crash. And so it is with some people in their prime, seemingly in excellent health, flying high, wide and handsome through life, feeling on top of the world, who may have a sudden flame-out—and a crash. A flame-out is always much more serious, dramatic and sudden than a "burn-out," and can involve a loss of life, loss of control over life, or just a serious loss of self-esteem. Men are far more likely to flame-out than women.

A common way to flame-out is by a heart attack. Thus we'll consider in depth the causes of, cures for, and ways of preventing heart attacks. Other major ways to flame-out are

3

by cancer, stroke, auto accident, drug overdose, or as a victim of violence. Another type of flame-out (reserved for men) is sexual impotence—a depressing experience, but not fatal.

With so many of our habits alleged to be bad by a variety of experts, how are we going to sort out which expert we are going to listen to? Failing to sort it out, we are most likely to try to forget it all, through a psychological process called denial. We'll just feel mildly guilty as we indulge our daily addictions—guilty that we may rob those who depend upon us by flaming out at a time when we appear to be in our prime.

Sometimes the experts contradict one another, and sometimes the facts contradict the experts. Let us consider some examples:

1. Smoking is considered an important risk factor in male heart disease. Yet where in the world do the men smoke the most cigarettes? In Japan, where they have by far the lowest rate of coronary heart disease of any industrialized country.

2. Exercise has been touted as a protection against heart disease. However, we hear of experienced marathoners dropping dead of a heart attack. Even the guru of running, Jim Fixx, succumbed at age 52. Tennis star Arthur Ashe certainly seemed to be fit when he suffered a heart attack at age 35. He survived it, and then joined the anti-cholesterol bandwagon.

3. Cholesterol has become the equivalent of the "bogeyman" in some circles. In ignorant fear, many fail to make the distinction between **dietary** cholesterol (found in some of our most nutritious foods) and **blood** cholesterol level. When the blood serum level of cholesterol is elevated above normal for a period of many years, there is an increased risk of coronary heart disease. It isn't often mentioned that most of the cholesterol in your bloodstream is manufactured by your own body, so that the problem of an elevated blood cholesterol level is primarily a problem of the body's regulation of it rather than one of dietary intake. Note the fact that dietary intake of cholesterol early in this century was very little different from the intake when coronary heart disease was at its peak in the 1960's. How can dietary cholesterol be

seriously considered as a cause of coronary heart disease?

4. Food fat is considered a major contributor to heart disease when consumed in excess. Americans consume 40 to 50 percent of their calories in food fat, and have a fairly high rate of heart disease. However, the Masai tribesmen of East Africa take in a whopping 65 percent of their calories in food fat, mostly saturated, but have almost no heart disease at any age. Saturated animal fat is the form usually accused of "clogging your arteries," but its consumption has changed little during this century in the U. S. A. If anything, it has gone down. Total fat consumption has been going up, even in recent years with coronary heart disease decreasing modestly. How can dietary fat be seriously considered as the culprit?

5. The idea of stress (type "A" behavior) as a cause of heart disease is continuing to grow in popularity. Stress is undoubtedly an important contributing factor in many cases, but can't be the whole story, since unstressed (type "B") individuals get heart attacks, too. Furthermore, stress heart attacks were certainly rare before this century, yet people had heavy stresses then, as now.

You have a perfect right to be confused. After all, the "facts" and the experts seem to disagree. While I could fill a whole book with the seeming contradictions from heart research, I won't because I know that you would like some useful answers. We'll get into the details shortly, but here I'll just mention that the key to understanding it all depends upon appreciating the many **interactions** that occur between the "bad habit" factors and certain nutritional factors.

We have to understand that most experts are narrow specialists, and tell you the conclusions they have reached from the data they have seen. Or perhaps an expert may be taking the word of some other more prestigious expert who may be on equally shaky scientific ground. With more data, they are likely to change their minds, unless they have a vested intellectual (or other) interest in the ideas. Additionally, the interpretation of scientific data, especially in the biomedical fields, is tricky. One never has all the data one wants, and it is difficult to know when there is sufficient data to reach firm conclusions.

The vast enterprise of medical and scientific research advances in a highly uncertain manner. Not only are there verbal battles between competing groups over ideas, but over who will get research funds. The best research ideas may not win out. Approaches are frequently taken that lose time and research funds without paying off. Ultimately, the right approach is found, but years or decades may be lost. But please don't give up on the scientific method, for it's still the best we have. Many heart researchers make the mistake of ignoring the field of nutritional biochemistry, a vast and rapidly growing body of knowledge, published in reputable biological-medical journals. While conventional thinking can never hope to make good progress against coronary heart disease, nutritional biochemical approaches may get close to eradicating it.

The scientists to be trusted the most are those with the broadest background training and experience, who are willing to spend years digging through mountains of data, constantly testing ideas and trying for an integration of the data of others. Such scientists are called generalists. Needless to say, there are never enough of that breed of scientist around, and there is no guarantee that the rest of the scientific community will listen to them. A generalist needs to be aloof from the various commercial vested interests, and have an independent source of financing.

I consider myself to be a generalist. I became determined to tackle the knotty problems of coronary heart disease eight years ago, after losing my two favorite relatives to it. Now I am able to explain the various strands of causation— and the measures needed for eradication.

CHAPTER 2

The Biggest Risks

Let us get to the real truth about your alleged bad habits, generally called risk factors. There is a **statistical** association between the risk factors and heart disease when we consider a sizeable group of Americans. But when we consider individuals, we can't use the risk factors to predict just who will get heart disease. Seemingly, many of you will get away with your bad habits. But some people, apparently with no bad habits, will get heart disease. It is clear that eliminating bad habits will only make a modest dent in the overall rate of heart disease. [Enloe '84, Kolata '85, Oliver '83] You will see that optimum nutrition is a much better approach to eliminating coronary heart disease.

You've heard the old saying about there being "lies, damn lies, and statistics." Statistical analysis has serious limitations, and can't yield scientific proof. In science, one has to regard statistical associations the same way as one regards "circumstantial evidence" in the field of law. The strength of a statistical association may tell us how likely or probable the connection between the events is. A very strong association suggests, but does not prove, a cause-effect relationship. But the associations between the risk factors and heart disease are not strong, and appear absent in some parts of the world, so that a cause-effect relationship is not particularly likely. While the risk factors are not causative, they do contribute in about the same way as the proverbial straw-that-broke-the-camel's-back.

Some adverse factors, other than the conventional risk

factors, are likely to be the main causes of heart disease. Most certainly, it is nothing new to suspect adverse factors in our modern diet. Many health educators, and part of the medical establishment, seem to push with almost religious zeal the idea that the important dietary risk factors are fat and cholesterol. Some other researchers, noting the problems with the fat-cholesterol hypothesis, are now discouraged in looking for **any** dietary factors. Clearly, we have to examine some other potentially adverse dietary factors.

There is good evidence that the modern civilized diet is a major cause—although a delayed cause—of heart attacks. Note that, as each isolated group of people gets exposed to outside commerce and gradually takes up the civilized diet, there is an increased incidence of many different health problems. In order of appearance, first comes tooth decay, then high blood pressure, later strokes, other circulatory problems, angina, and finally heart attacks. The time span over which these diseases make their appearance is about 30 years. [Trowell '81; Wadsworth '84]

Looking at the Western "civilized" life of past centuries, we find heart attacks rather rare. Coronary heart disease was first identified in the 1700's, but was not medically diagnosed until the late 1800's. [McGee '79] It began a steep rise in incidence after 1920. [Anderson '73; Stallones '80] Perhaps, though, some who died of "apoplexy" or "acute indigestion" earlier may actually have had heart attacks. At any rate, the incidence of coronary heart disease in the middle-age brackets would seem to have multiplied at least ten times from the last century to this one.

The situation of the modern American looks far worse when compared to someone from a culture that hasn't been converted to modern food technology. Just consider that an American is about 3,000 times as likely to get a heart attack as one of the mountain people of Dagestan in the Russian Caucasus. [Benet '76] I deliberately choose to compare an American to someone in a culture in which the people are white, where they eat eggs and red meat heartily, and smoke tobacco or ferment the grape, but in whom heart attacks are rare. One could choose from other cultures with low rates of heart attack, but it is best to have a comparison with a culture that uses the same basic foodstuffs (although unmodified). In case some researchers argue that the Dagestan people haven't been studied thoroughly enough, I can fall back upon the example of the Masai, who are different racially and in many habits, but have been thoroughly studied. [Biss '71; Day '76; Gibney '80; Ho '71; Mann '72, '64] There are many other peoples around the world who are virtually free of heart disease, making it clear that we don't need to suffer from it. [Lowenstein '64; McGee '79]

It makes the most sense to compare Americans to meat, fat, and cholesterol-eating peoples who have no coronary heart disease—for this helps cancel out the misconceptions fostered by some "experts," who seem to be fond of comparing Americans to vegetarian peoples, and then coming up with the unwarranted idea that we have to give up eating meat, fat and cholesterol to eliminate heart disease.

Let us say that the average American has two bad habits more than someone from the Caucasus mountains. Then, if each bad habit multiplies the risk of a heart attack by three, which is roughly correct for the worst bad habits like stress and smoking, the American would be nine times (3 x 3) as likely to have a heart attack. If there are interactions (synergism) between the two bad habits, the risk could conceivably be multiplied by thirty. Whatever, you wouldn't expect heart attack risks to be multiplied by 3,000 because of a couple of slightly bad habits. Thus "unknown" factors push the figure up by at least 100 times, and those factors are very likely something in the diet, since we've researched the hell out of all other possible factors and no others could account for it.

Evidence for factors in the modern civilized diet (other than fat and cholesterol) being the biggest risk factors behind coronary heart disease is discussed in detail in later chapters, where several specific dietary risk factors—and protective factors—are evaluated. Previous difficulties in sorting out dietary risk factors occurred because not all of the interacting factors were examined together in any one statistical study.

I have been able to display the interacting factors graphically using data from other researchers. It turns out that there are injurious factors in milk which will act when there are not enough of the protective factors found in whole grains and vegetables. (Note: the term "vegetables" includes salads.) Surprisingly, there are strongly protective factors in fermented milk products, such as in yogurt and cheese. Two other damaging factors, salt and fat, can also contribute to coronary heart disease. Amazingly, milk fat appears much less injurious than something present in the skim milk fraction. (See Chapter 7 for details on these interacting factors.)

But how drastic are the changes needed in your diet? The answer depends upon a number of factors. It depends upon whether you are male or female, how long you've been eating the all-American diet, how many health problems you've already developed, your genetic make-up, how much pollution you are exposed to, and how many of the so-called bad habits you indulge in. The more of these factors going against you, the more likely your body's regulation and self-repair mechanisms are functioning poorly, and the greater your need for super quality food plus certain vitamin and mineral supplements. For the average person, the changes needed are not drastic—and require no real sacrifice. Men need to be more cautious than women.

To sum it up, you need to switch from fluid milk to yogurt and cheese, and from refined grains and sugars to whole grains and starches. As additional protection, you could also get more vegetables and salads and ease off a bit on salt and fat—advisable especially for those who have a family history of heart disease. Many Americans also need more of an oil called "EPA" (explained later). Following this advice, I estimate you can reduce your chances of a heart attack by 90 percent. If you add on vitamin and mineral supplementation tailored to individual needs, the chances would be reduced by 99 percent.

It appears that we were brainwashed to believe in the importance of the conventional risk factors, when actually the main heart risks are in the modern civilized diet.

Let us now look at some of the hazards of being a man.

CHAPTER 3

Helping Men Live Longer

With women outliving men by over seven years, it appears that the current approach to male health needs a thorough overhaul.

It is not difficult to identify the reasons for the difference in life expectancy. Men have the dubious distinction of leading in all major categories of causes of death. Men are far more likely to die from accidents or violence, or in wars——perhaps reflecting the more aggressive and venturesome nature that is associated with males. More men than women die of cancer, especially of lung cancer among smokers. More men die of liver cirrhosis, a special hazard among heavy drinkers. Many more men are successful at suicide, though more women attempt it. But it is coronary heart disease that shortens average male life span the most.

This mass killer of men appeared during this century, rising from obscurity before 1920 to being a major epidemic from the 1950's until now. In 1920, heart disease claimed about as many women as men, but the predominant modern form, **coronary** heart disease, thrives on a special vulnerability of men. [Anderson '73] It selectively kills men in their middle years——25 times as many men as women in some parts of Europe, but more like 7 times in the U.S. figures. Now you know why there are five times as many widows as widowers.

There have been charges coming from some women's groups that a male-dominated medical profession gives women rather insensitive medical care. No doubt the women have a reasonable complaint, but it would seem that men have more to complain about. The primary medical specialist for women tends to be the gynecologist, while that for men would appear to be the coroner or the cardiologist. Let's hope that no psychiatrist will suggest that men have a death wish.

Throughout history, men have died a few years younger than women, but only during the most ruinous wars has the male/female difference in life expectancy approached a figure of the proportions of today. Some of the reason has to do with a man's hormones, which make him (on average) more aggressive and adventurous than women. Thus men have had a greater predilection for wars and risky ventures, and get into violent scrapes more often. Many men have an illusion of invincibility or immortality, especially when young and feisty. We could call it the Alexander-the-Great syndrome. There is an excess of self-confidence, and of macho or bravado. Sometimes that helps a man get through trouble and win out (similar to the instinct for dominance in male animals), but it can also get him in worse trouble.

Wisdom consists in a man fortifying himself with all possible knowledge. Then he can take reasonable, calculated risks, in which he knows the odds are in his favor, especially when the potential benefits are great. For a man's lifelong good health, be assured that wisdom lies in appreciating the importance of certain nutritional factors, and worrying less about the conventional risk factors.

The male hormone testosterone does not help men live longer. In medieval times, when some males were castrated at a tender age, either to preserve a beautiful singing voice or for tending harems, it was found that eunuchs on average lived longer than normal men. But who would want to be castrated to live a bit longer? It's the quality of life that most concerns us, not the years lived. Yet what is a popular type of drug that doctors use in trying to bring down high blood pressure or prevent a second heart attack? It's called a "beta-blocker" and it helps keep you from reacting quite as strongly to outside stimuli. As a side effect, some men will lose interest in sex or be unable to get an erection—no longer able to respond to the charms of a warm and willing woman. What man wants this sort of drug approach for extending his life?   Certainly, life would **seem** longer.

One key to increasing male life expectancy, and improving the quality of life in the later years, lies in raising male consciousness of the importance of certain nutritional factors. (Wives/mates can help here.)   While there have been some definite improvements in nutrition during this century, some other dietary changes have produced nutritional imbalances that happen to negatively affect male longevity much more than female longevity.

But first we must dispose of the prevalent idea that coronary heart disease is the result of people living longer. You've all heard that average life spans in the U. S. A. and northern European countries have been rising steadily.   The main reason lies in the reduction of the death rates for women, babies and small children.   The middle-aged man has gained little in life expectancy.   A fifty year old male today can look forward to only a few extra years of life over a man in Colonial times.   Can you guess in which countries a 45-year old male has the greatest number of years of life remaining? The answer: Greece, Costa Rica and Cuba—with 31.5 years left to live.   [Sinclair '82]

We have a sizeable bulge in male death rates from the age of 45 and up.   In previous centuries, death rates did not vary as much with age, for infectious diseases carried people off at any age.   Could it be that the younger men now spared from dying of infectious diseases are the same ones who are dying in their 40's and 50's of coronary heart disease and other degenerative diseases?   I seriously doubt it, for there doesn't appear to be much connection between these two vastly different life threats.   Men seem to have traded one life threat (infectious diseases in earlier times) for another (modern degenerative diseases), and gained little of life span in the trade.   It is difficult to imagine how men get coronary heart disease because of living longer, although this probably applies for a small proportion of men.

With the world's greatest technology, why can't we do a better job of keeping men alive in their middle years?   I am firmly convinced that the medical research establishment needs a **new conceptual framework** in which to think of male health and heart disease. With a better conceptual framework, rapid progress can be made in eradicating coronary heart disease——helping men to live longer. The new framework must be based heavily upon nutritional biochemical knowledge, which is the foundation for nutritional therapy. (I've made an attempt in this direction in Appendix I.)

Nutritional therapy——improving/modifying the diet and using vitamin and mineral supplements——can help far more than drugs. Nutritional therapy has few adverse side effects. In fact, it frequently has beneficial side effects, like curing more health problems than the therapist was trying to cure. As an example of how nutritional therapy can save lives, consider some research work of James P. Isaacs, M. D. He had available 25 people who had had one or more heart attacks and who were failing under the conventional cardiology treatment of the 1960's. He gave them balanced nutritional supplements which included both vitamins and minerals. (Also included was a modest dose of thyroid hormone.) Of the 21 men in the program, 19 were alive and well 10 years later and had had no further heart attacks. Of the two men lost, one died soon after the program began, when he returned too quickly to a job that required physical exertion. The other quit the supplements after six years, developed angina, and then died of a heart attack while doctors were using invasive procedures to examine his arteries. [Isaacs '71] Perhaps both deaths were unnecessary, and would not happen now with the latest knowledge of both nutritional therapy and conventional cardiology treatment. It indicates how much the coronary patient's life can hang in the balance and be tipped over by small events.

The 90% survival rate for the men in Isaac's study was remarkable, especially considering the fact that the patients were chosen because they were failing after their heart attacks. During the nutritional therapy, the men had other health improvements, such as greater exercise tolerance, better skin texture and appearance, reduced problems with teeth and gums, etc. All symptoms of heart disease disappeared. If nutritional therapy had not been used, probably less than half the men would have survived, and the survivors might have led a rather limited life.

Their survival and thriving under nutritional therapy was not just a chance event happening with a modest number of cases. To see this, try flipping a coin 21 times, and most likely it will come up with heads 10 or 11 times, comparable to the expected number of survivors with conventional treatment. You would have to keep repeating the set of 21 flips day in and day out for a month (maybe 5000 times) before you would by chance get as many as 19 out of 21 flips coming up heads, representing chance survival of 19 of the 21 men—a very unlikely event. But still, the number of cases was small, so Dr. Isaacs took on 100 new cases, treating them for a longer period of time. The results don't appear to be available as yet.

Let us compare Isaac's excellent nutritional therapy results to the meagre results of drug trials in expensive research projects. Results in 1981 showed that beta-blocking drugs can reduce the incidence of second heart attacks by 30%. In 1984, it was shown that a drug that lowers blood cholesterol could reduce heart attacks 20% in **high risk** males. [LRC '84; Nutrition Today '84] I emphasize "high risk" because it won't necessarily do anything for the average male. Besides, among the men getting the drug, there was an alarming number of men dying in accidents or suicide, or developing cancer.

The comparable figure on the reduction of second heart attacks by using nutritional therapy, based upon Dr. Isaacs work, would be 80% (or higher, depending upon how the data is handled). On top of that, nutritional therapy had beneficial side effects, whereas the drug therapies had annoying side effects. It is distressing to see excellent nutritional therapy results forgotten, and later buried by media hype about drug approaches that are comparatively ineffective. [Enloe '84] The latest nutritional therapy, individualized for the patient and carried out by an M. D. of the nutritional specialty, could virtually eliminate second heart attacks.

If nutritional therapy can cure heart trouble in those who have already had a heart attack, it should certainly be able to prevent heart attacks in those who have never had one. Prevention is certainly the best strategy. It only requires modest changes in diet, plus vitamin and mineral supplements.

CHAPTER 4

Staying Out of Trouble

You may have noted that I ended the last chapter with a pitch for prevention of health problems. Of course, everyone extols prevention. But why don't we practice it more often?

One of the major reasons may be that we have difficulty perceiving a cause-effect relationship when the effect lags the cause by time periods greater than a few days. The classic case might be that of vitamin C and scurvy. It takes a month or two for someone to come down with scurvy after prime vitamin C food sources are removed. It took the British about 500 years to find out why sailors got scurvy and then another 200 years to convince the British Admiralty to adopt the necessary measures. The Yukon Indians may have done better at it, for they discovered that they could get a health-preserving effect by removing and dividing up among their hunting group the freshly removed adrenal glands (which are rich in vitamin C) of the animals they bagged. We have no idea how long it took them to solve that nutritional problem. In the case of other health problems related to inadequate nutrition, the time periods for development of maladies may vary from days to decades, so that seeing (or proving for the skeptics) the cause-effect relationship is most difficult.

Another hindrance to the practice of prevention is the illusion of invincibility, probably more of a problem with men than women. A feeling of self-confidence and of being "lucky" can do us in. We have the tendency to think that it's always the other person who gets in trouble. I am no better than the rest of you, for in my early forties, I suddenly realized that I had a dozen different annoying health complaints, and started to ask, "Why me?" Fortunately, a friend happened to toss a nutrition book at me. Honestly, before that, even with excellent graduate school training in the biological/medical sciences, I blindly missed seeing the connections between biochemistry and the food going into my mouth. I foolishly believed the assurances of government officials as to the adequacy of the all-American diet, and thought that my good genes would insure a long, healthy life.

It was over a period of many years of much study that I eliminated most of my health problems through improved diet, experimenting to find the supplements that my body needed in extra amounts, and identifying some food allergies. After losing my father and my uncle to heart disease, I dove into intensive study of books and medical journal articles on the subject, and did my own thinking.

Over the same span of time, the field of nutritional therapy has also been developing. Along the way, I met many other people who had been let down by conventional medical practice, and found that many of them could also be helped by nutritional therapy. It is unfortunate that doctors get very little training in nutrition in medical school. Thus they miss out on some of the better ways of helping many of their patients. (Doctors will find it hard to believe the incredible numbers of great research articles on nutrition published in a wide variety of medical journals. Many of these journals are cited in the Reference Notes.)

Also working against the practice of prevention are the addictions that we acquire to the many readily available taste-tempting treats and seductive sweets. Surprisingly, some of the foods to which we get addicted are ones that we are allergic to. You'll see later that we have some innate tastes that lead us astray, and thus there is a need for self-discipline. Let's face it, we are all weak in some ways—but let's resolve to be weak only in the things that aren't so important. There are more interesting and less hazardous vices available than the all-American diet.

Another hindrance to prevention is a fatalistic argument that we sometimes hear. Let's say that your father and your grandfather died young of heart disease. Thus you fully expect to do the same, and think that there is nothing you can do about it. Totally wrong! Certainly you may be a genetic type that is susceptible to coronary heart disease, but I very much doubt that your great-grandfather died young of coronary heart disease, because the disease was rare back then. There are probably a number of different genetic factors that raise susceptibility to coronary heart disease, but all should be treatable by specific nutritional therapies. If you are at risk, it is all the more reason to be nutritionally cautious. Superior nutrition and the right vitamin and mineral supplements will help protect you from disability or an early grave.

A further important hindrance to the practice of prevention is that a heart attack can seem to strike with no warning at all. I know one fellow who always feels great, even before each of the heart attacks he has had. Some have a feeling of unusual fatigue beforehand. [Guerci '80] However, such a feeling is most definitely not a specific warning sign. Don't forget that only half of those who have a heart attack get a chance to correct their nutrition. The other half end up on a slab at the coroner's.

Let's consider for a few moments the alternatives to prevention. There are all kinds of medical heroics that have been developed to help you if you get a heart attack. If you don't suffer sudden cardiac death, you'll live for the crowds gathering, the screaming sirens, cardiopulmonary resuscitation, the emergency room, the hospital bed, all the flowers your friends will send (if not placed on your casket), various needles stuck in you, all kinds of blinking lights on the electronic monitors, possible coronary bypass operation, a long convalescence, huge hospital bills and doctor fees, possibly having to give up your job permanently, stern warnings from your physician about the way you live your life, constant worry as to when the next attack might come, worry as to whether you should indulge in sex anymore, . . . By now, you've certainly heard too much about life after a heart attack.

If you get into trouble, don't expect to be rescued by a coronary bypass operation, a heart transplant or an artificial heart, for:

1. A coronary bypass operation will be helpful to some, but, for the long term, those who get the operation must also improve their nutrition to maintain the benefits. It is far better to improve your nutrition now, so that you never get into a desperate situation.

2. Only one heart patient in a thousand gets a chance at a heart transplant, and even then long term survival is not assured. There are horrendous problems with the body trying to reject the "foreign" tissue of the new heart. (Note that any nutritional therapy must be avoided that might strengthen the immune system.)

3. There will never be an artificial heart as good as the one Mother Nature designed for you. Just consider that your own heart and circulatory system has built into it all sorts of self-repair and feedback-control systems, which involve nerve connections and chemical messengers (i. e., hormones and prostaglandins). You can't expect an artificial heart to interface well with the other parts of your system, nor can you expect the artificial heart to repair itself. In those who have received an artificial heart so far, there are an alarming number of strokes occurring.

* * *

Seeing these appalling alternatives to prevention, it is hoped that you'll resolve to practice prevention diligently. The first step to transcending all the previously-mentioned hindrances to prevention is to recognize and accept them. Then, one must apply a bit of self-discipline.

The message is: Keep your own heart in good repair by providing it with all the nutritional factors it needs. Then you'll probably never need medical heroics practiced on you.

CHAPTER 5

Man Muddles Through

It is amazing that people who wouldn't think of putting the wrong kind of fuel in their cars don't hesitate to put any old kind of food-fuel into their mouths.   It is more astonishing that we breed our animals mostly on excellent food-fuels, making it into a science.   Then industrialized people ignore science and eat all sorts of heavily advertised, high-tech food—as if mankind were an exception to the laws of life. Without the proper food-fuels, your system will develop some subtle and some not-so-subtle ailments.   Just as trying to operate a jet engine on the wrong fuel can cause it to flame-out, so can the wrong food-fuels lead you to a flame-out.   Of course, in your case, there is likely to be a longer time lag.

In engineering terms, 'Homo sapiens' is an excellent design, but can't be expected to run well on inappropriate fuel. Our mind/body system will operate best mostly on the food-fuels on which mankind evolved.   Thus, to better understand optimum nutrition, we must take into account the evolutionary development of mankind.

We evolved over a period of many millions of years, but our biochemistry is probably not much different from our precursors, the mammals.   The foods that are most suited to our body's needs are the ones that were eaten during that early development period.   These foods must have included primarily meat, fish, fowl, fruits, berries, various leafy and root vegetables, and wild grains.   We'll call this the **primitive diet.**   Some, mostly isolated, peoples around the world still have this type of "hunter-gatherer" diet.

20

The domestication of animals for meat and milk, and the cultivation of grains, were comparatively recent developments that took place possibly 10 to 15 thousand years ago. Not surprisingly, some people's bodies try to reject these more recent additions to our diet as if the foods were an enemy invasion. Bad reactions occur most frequently with milk or with the most commonly used grains, wheat and corn. There can be allergies, coming on in a half hour with almost any symptom; or a food sensitivity (possibly a delayed response), typically with a persistent belly ache; or a cerebral allergy with psychological or behavioral symptoms; or a food intolerance, in which digestion and absorption of nutrients are disrupted by the offending food. With milk, the cleverness of our ancestors led to cheeses and yogurt, which kept without refrigeration, and tended to cause many fewer bad reactions.

As an example of an ancient diet that helped produce super athletes, we might consider that of the contenders in the Olympic games of the sixth to the eighth century B. C. Some of these super athletes had careers that spanned decades. They competed and won year after year, even though entered in many different events. Their typical food included very coarse bread, barley cakes (with a bit of milk, oil, or honey in the dough), figs, cherries, olives, goat cheese (Feta cheese), modest amounts of goat or deer meat (occasionally beef), and wine. Salt was also important, but used far less than today. Several centuries later, Olympic athletes were devouring huge quantities of beef. But they must have lacked endurance, for they did not tend to compete year after year. The earlier, highly successful Olympic diet bears considerable resemblance to the latest high complex-carbohydrate diets recommended for athletes.

Until this past century, our foods were only modified in fairly simple ways. The refinement of sugar and grains has been known for the past several thousand years, but took place on a small scale, since only the wealthy could afford to indulge. With the industrial revolution and the development of powerful machines, it became possible to modify foods on a mass scale and to do it at low cost. Mass agriculture and food distribution systems also came into being. Villages grew into cities, and cities became metropolises, with the proportion of people in an urban environment increasing. However, don't yearn for "the good old days." We may hate the automobile with its hazards of pollution, noise and accidents, but consider how New Yorkers felt at the beginning of this century. They looked forward to the automobile as giving blessed relief from all the smelly horse manure in the streets, and from the incredible number of flies that bred in it.

We have benefited from all these changes in many ways, but have unwittingly become experimental "guinea pigs." The technologists overseeing the changes believed they were doing good, but didn't usually have a broad enough perspective to foresee possible adverse effects. The refinement of grains, with removal of the bran and germ, was a particularly bad change, for it causes the partial or complete loss of about two dozen different nutrients, giving rise to complex nutritional imbalances. But not all food processing should be condemned, for foods such as milk and soybeans both undergo important improvements during processing.

There is really no possibility of, or benefit in, returning to the conditions of the primitive world. After all, primitive life was (and is) rough. However, we should try to approach the primitive type diet. Average life span in primitives tends to be short because of high death rates among children under age four. Infectious diseases, resulting mainly from poor sanitation, add somewhat to the death rates at all ages. But primitive people lack the degenerative diseases that afflict Western man, and some individuals among them live to ripe old ages. In primitive and less-developed societies, male death rates in the 45 to 70 age bracket tend to be much lower than those in Western culture——mainly because there is no coronary heart disease.

Because we are all different genetically, it will be found that some can safely depart from the primitive foods more than others. An immediate bad reaction from a food tells us what we have to do——avoid it. But if the "bad reactions" are in the form of degenerative diseases that take years or decades to express themselves, there is no easy way to sort out the foods that are bad for us.

Let us look briefly at how nutritional science developed. The spurs to the early development of nutritional science were certain deficiency diseases.   The refinement of grains in the past century helped people in warm humid climates to store grains (such as rice) or flours (wheat and corn) longer without weevil infestations, but led to human diseases like beri-beri and pellagra.   With the limited nutritional knowledge earlier in this century, it was found that the addition of a few vitamins seemed to prevent the problems.   Because owners of the machinery had large investments and people had new-found tastes for white flour, white rice, and degerminated corn meal, the addition of a few vitamins seemed to be the appropriate solution.   Thus, people did not go back to using whole grains, for the "experts" of that period thought it was sufficient to add a few vitamins to refined grains.

Of course, at that time, it wasn't realized that there were a whole slew of undiscovered beneficial food factors that were being lost by this jury-rigged solution.   Many of these more recently discovered nutrients do not tend to become depleted from the body until after months or even years of inadequate intake.   The result can be insidious degenerative diseases making an appearance decades later.   Because people vary in their abilities to absorb or retain nutrients, some may escape the problems.   But who wants to be the one to gamble and take the risks?   Natural selection might be working— against you.   Thus it is safest to use whole grains—whole grain bread rather than white bread, brown rice instead of white rice, and whole corn meal instead of degerminated corn meal.   We are no longer constrained by a limited shelf life, for we have refrigerators, freezers, and can also grind our own grains fresh using an inexpensive grinder.   There are other nutritional benefits of whole grains, such as from the fiber, which helps keep your gut working right, helps in control of blood cholesterol levels, and helps prevent colon cancer in people on high fat diets.

Some primitive diets must have had a good mix of nutrients, especially when a wide variety of foods were consumed.   But a wide variety of foods is not a guarantee, for in many parts of the world the soils are depleted of certain mineral nutrients. Glaciated areas are missing minerals such as iodine (needed to prevent goiter), selenium, sulfur, and zinc. Tropical rain forests tend to be short in calcium, magnesium and many trace minerals, because the rains leach minerals out of the soil. At one time, New Zealand soil was missing cobalt, and the grasses wouldn't support cattle and sheep until the problem was corrected.

While some of the human tribes must have thrived, others barely survived with a life that would seem miserable to us. The rare ones that achieved optimum nutrition and optimum health generally lived in mountainous areas. Some reasons for this could be that, with dolomitic rock, the water is very hard, full of calcium, magnesium and probably trace elements as well. In the mountains, the air tends to be clean and loaded with health-promoting negative ions. Sanitation is not a problem, for the lowlands get the effluvia. Overcrowding is less likely to happen.

Mankind's animal ancestors, the mammals, evolved in a rather unfriendly environment. You may wonder, how did these creatures survive, having far less brain capacity than we have? It is apparent that they gradually evolved a large number of **protective mechanisms,** which aided them in their climb up out of the slime. There is no other way to explain survival of this line of animals. As part of our animal heritage, we retained many of these protective mechanisms.

As our first example, consider that our bodies have mechanisms for detoxifying various poisons. You may be horrified to learn that many of our everyday foods contain natural toxins unrelated to those that man has added. Some vegetables may have evolved toxins to protect from insect infestations. Fortunately, we have learned to avoid the most toxic plants (or parts of plants). By getting variety in our foods, we can avoid getting overloaded by toxins in any one food. Some vegetable toxins are eliminated by soaking, cooking, or other processing. The remaining mild toxins are taken care of by our detoxifying mechanisms, located mainly in the liver. The mechanisms can also handle a certain amount of environmental pollutants. (Drugs that we take are also detoxified.) But our detoxifying mechanisms do have their limits—frequently exceeded in our modern environment. If on some days you feel lousy, maybe its because you got too much poison. There are also drastic differences between individuals in their tolerance for toxins. Note well that optimum nutrition and supplements can help keep your detoxifying mechanisms working at their peak.

As another example of a protective mechanism, your body has abilities to regulate the absorption, retention, or excretion of mineral nutrients. Thus your body can handle a range of intakes. If you don't get enough of a particular mineral nutrient, as would occur if you eat many refined foods, your body does its best to absorb or retain it better. But there are limits to the body's adaptive mechanisms. When your body tries to increase absorption of a mineral, toxic metals will be inadvertently pulled in as well. Thus, inadequate calcium intake contributes to lead uptake, inadequate magnesium contributes to aluminum uptake, and inadequate zinc or selenium intake contributes to cadmium, mercury, or arsenic uptake.

The means that man has for storing many nutrients in his body tend to help him in times of famine. But he wasn't designed for modern foods that have many calories and minimal nutrients. On these foods, the body tends to get depleted of many nutrients over a period of time, and toxic metal absorption is encouraged. What tends to lose out are many of the body's regulatory and self-repair mechanisms, contributing to the development of degenerative diseases decades later.

You can appreciate the body's need for maintenance and self-repair mechanisms if you consider that your heart beats about three billion times during your lifetime, and that arteries and other tissues are stretched with each beat. Can you imagine any inanimate material being able to withstand that many flexures without fatiguing and breaking? The best inanimate materials can only be flexed about ten million times before breaking. That is only 1/300 of the flexings in your circulatory system. If you let your own system deteriorate, you can't expect any adequate man-made replacements. In the word "atherosclerosis," the prefix "athero" means "mush." You can keep your innards from turning to mush by providing your body with adequate amounts of all the necessary repair materials, that is, the **essential nutrients.** (See next chapter.)

Among his protective mechanisms, man has some innate tastes for food. [Kare '75] These innate tastes would have aided his survival in primitive times. But in the modern environment, some of these same tastes lead him astray. For example, there are innate tastes for salt, fat, sugar, and perhaps the feel of smooth foods in the mouth. These tastes would have had survival value in the primitive inland environment. Salt is especially scarce in inland areas, and even the kidney mechanisms for conserving sodium reflect this fact. Fat would also have been scarce in the primitive environment, and a taste for it would guide us to high grade animal or plant proteins, as well as to a concentrated energy source. A sweet taste would guide us to carbohydrates, providing calories that are well packaged with vitamins, minerals, and fiber. A desire to feel smooth foods in the mouth would have helped us avoid eating woody, indigestible materials that could cause choking or other blockage. Adding complexity to the scientific issues is the fact that our tastes tend to become distorted when modern foods deplete nutrients from our bodies.

In our modern environment, innate tastes have helped lead us into excess, aided and abetted by our ingenuity in breaking apart foods through modern food technology. The food technologists are merely catering to our tastes. Our main defense against innate tastes leading us astray lies in self-discipline, bolstered by a knowledge of our inherited weaknesses. You can help cause the worst of these foods to disappear from the market place if you stop buying them.

It is apparent that man has survived most of his history by just muddling through, aided by many built-in protective mechanisms. But now he is led astray by certain of these mechanisms—the innate tastes mentioned. It is time for him to apply his enlarged brain to the problems at hand.

One advantage of getting a variety of primitive type foods in your diet is that you won't need to know quite as much about nutrition to stay in good health. However, I hope to educate you in that subject anyway. Let us start with some nutritional chemistry.

CHAPTER 6

The Chemistry of Life

You are incredibly complex, with many aspects of your chemistry only partly understood. However, using only simple chemistry, I can show you how nutrition fits into the chemistry of living things, and how living systems are organized. You'll then understand better the many nutritional terms that you've heard tossed around for so many years.

The chemical reactions of life take place in watery surroundings. By weight, you are nearly 3/4 water, much of it liquid, but part of the water is tightly or loosely bound with the molecules of life. About 1/5 of body weight is in organic chemical compounds—molecules, or combinations of molecules forming structures. The mineral content of your body is about 1/25 of your weight, mostly the calcium and phosphorus in your bones. Only a fraction of the minerals are in a water solution as ions or other loosely-bound chemical forms, but this small fraction is vital for your body's normal chemical reactions.

While there is a structure of cells, tissues and organs, let us first look far below these levels to that of molecules and chemical events. The molecules of life are chain and ring structure compounds, mostly with a backbone of carbon atoms but occasionally with a nitrogen or sulfur atom substituted into the backbone. Onto the atoms of the backbone are attached atoms of hydrogen, or oxygen, or nitrogen, or sulfur, or combinations of these. The main classes of molecules are proteins, carbohydrates, lipids and nucleic acids. Many are huge "macromolecules" containing many thousands of atoms.

It is the arrangements and interactions of all these

different molecules and ions in the watery matrix that are of interest.   There are complex networks of chemical reactions taking place, step by step, in specific locations, with perhaps 10,000 different chemical reactions taking place at the same time.   The sum total of all these chemical processes occurring is called the metabolism.   The building up of molecules in the body is called anabolism, and the breaking down of molecules, for getting rid of them or for gaining energy, is called catabolism.   The body's tissues are constantly being built and rebuilt, part of the process of maintenance and self-repair.

These chemical reactions are aided by enzymes, which are mostly protein molecules that act as biological catalysts. The enzymes allow the chemical reactions to proceed rapidly at body temperature.   We still talk about "burning" food for energy, measured in kilocalories, but always called "Calories" (with a capital "C") by nutritionists.   If you take in and burn 2500 Calories per day, then your heat output will be about 100 watts.   Carbohydrates and fats end up mostly as carbon dioxide and water, just as if flamed at a high temperature. Proteins are not broken down as completely.

Most of these enzymes are manufactured in the cells of your body, under instructions coded in your genetic material by nucleic acids, which are in the form of long chains twisted into a double helix.   For functioning, the enzymes usually require co-enzymes, and/or cofactors.   Many of the mineral ions act as cofactors.   The enzymes or co-enzymes that your body needs, but can't manufacture itself, are called vitamins. Vitamins you must get from your food or supplements.

We can think of vitamins as facilitators of the body's normal chemical reactions.   In contrast, pharmaceutical drugs are mostly inhibitors of chemical reactions.   Usually, drugs will inhibit in more places than desired, giving rise to side effects.   In normal dosages, vitamins have no side effects, but some have adverse side effects at high doses.   [Miller '82] Some vitamin enthusiasts never mention side effects, whereas some skeptics about vitamins only mention the possible side effects, omitting mention of beneficial effects.   I hope to give a balanced view.

When I've used the term mineral, your first thought could

have been about rock crystals or aggregates that geologists concern themselves with. Your bones are the only part of your body that fit the geologist's definition of mineral. But the way nutritional science developed, the term mineral came to be applied to all the chemical elements that are found to be essential to living things (except the elements of the carbon chain or ring molecules). Most of the minerals are metallic elements, but some are non-metallic. These minerals in the body will exist in the form of ions in solution (electrolyte minerals) or combined loosely or tightly by various types of chemical bonds. When in the form of a loosely bound metal ion that can be transferred easily to another bound form, it is apt to be called a chelate (pronounced "key-late"). Chelated mineral supplements are usually absorbed better in the gut.

We talk about macrominerals, the ones needed in large quantities by your body, and about trace minerals (preferably called trace elements), the ones needed in tiny quantities (less than 1 part in 10,000 in your diet). [Mertz '84, '83, '81, '80; Shamberger '80]

The essential nutrients include these minerals, plus vitamins, essential amino acids, and essential fatty acids. There are some 50 to 60 essential nutrients. "Essential" is becoming a fuzzy term because there are genetic differences in people's abilities to manufacture substances the body needs. The number can not be fixed as yet because new ones could be discovered. Also, the essentiality of some nutrients is controversial. Nutrition researchers like to discover new ones. It is one way to get ahead in the professional world but colleagues may be reluctant to agree that the vitamin exists, or that the vitamin or mineral is essential, or that the researcher has provided sufficient proof. Some controversial nutrients may not be essential for life but may be needed for optimum health, at least by some people.

Among the generally accepted vitamins, we have A, B, C, D, E, and K, where B includes the B-complex factors of B-1 (thiamine), B-2 (riboflavin), B-3 (niacin, nicotinic acid, or niacinamide), B-5 (pantothenic acid), B-6 (pyridoxine), B-12 (cobalamin), biotin, and folic acid. Somewhat less accepted as essential are choline, inositol, and PABA (paraaminobenzoic

acid).   Among some other candidates as B-complex vitamins
are lipoic acid and B-13 (orotic acid).   Pangamic acid, a
useful supplement to aid tissue oxygenation and stimulate the
immune system, is sometimes called vitamin B-15, but is not
strictly a vitamin except in Russia.   A highly controversial
one is B-17 (laetrile or amygdalin), used by some in cancer
therapy, but whose efficacy is much in doubt.   L-carnitine is
a non-vitamin nutrient needed in the burning of fat.   It is rich
in meat and also produced adequately in most people's bodies.

Researchers have nearly used up the entire alphabet with
proposed vitamins.   Thus in some books you may find vitamin F
(essential fatty acids), vitamin P (bioflavonoids), and even Q
and U, but the chemical names are preferred.   One advantage
of eating a variety of whole foods is that you have a better
chance of getting all the vitamins and minerals, including the
ones that haven't been discovered or accepted as yet.

One group of minerals that are of great importance to
your health are the ones that form electrolyte ions: calcium,
magnesium, sodium, potassium, and chlorine (as chloride).
Calcium and magnesium are also of vital importance in more
tightly bound chemical complexes.   Phosphorus is another
mineral of considerable importance and quantity and is always
in the phosphate form.   Sulfur is an important mineral that is
generally part of an amino acid, but some is present in the
sulfate form.

The most vital trace elements are zinc, copper, iron,
chromium, manganese, selenium, and iodine (as iodide).   None
of the metallic elements is used as a metal.   They exist only in
the charged state in which they have lost electrons.   In the
case of chromium, the form with a +3 valence (i.e., it has given
away 3 electrons in going from the neutral metallic state) is
vital to life, whereas the form with a +6 valence, as in
industrial chromates, is a poison.   Chromium is most useful as
part of the GTF (glucose tolerance factor) molecule, being
therapeutic for hypoglycemics.   Cobalt is also essential in
man but only as part of the vitamin B-12 molecule.   Excesses
of the trace elements become toxic.

Some other trace elements that appear essential are
bromine, fluorine, molybdenum, nickel, silicon, vanadium and

tin. Even arsenic is essential in the minute quantity of 0.1 ppm (parts per million). Lithium and rubidium would not be considered essential but have beneficial effects in some circumstances: lithium in psychiatric disorders and rubidium in cancer protection.

One thing about many minerals is that the range of safe dosage is much narrower than that for vitamins. Also, there are many **interferences** between minerals, that is, too much of one will adversely affect absorption or body levels of another. Good mineral supplementation may require several separate pills, because of both bulkiness and interferences between different minerals. Vitamins, except for large doses of C, take up little space, and easily fit into one pill.

Proteins are long chains of amino acid molecules joined together by what is called a peptide bond, which gives a strand of protein a helical form (like a coil spring). There are almost an infinite number of possible protein molecules that can exist, since every protein may have hundreds of amino acids strung together in a chain, and each amino acid along the chain could be any one of 22 different amino acids. Many of your protein molecules are unique to yourself and your close relatives, created under the instructions of your genes, but they may differ from those of other people in only a few amino acids out of a hundred. The backbone of a protein molecule may be coiled up into a ball (globule) because of electrical charges on the individual amino acids that make up the protein, or protein molecules may be layered together by these same electrical attraction forces to form structural parts of the body. Protein enzymes will have "hot spots," or locations at which the proximity of another reactant will cause a specific chemical reaction to take place.

When we eat proteins, they are broken down in our gut into short chains of amino acids by stomach acids and digestive enzymes. In the small intestine they are further broken down into individual amino acids. If your body doesn't break down proteins sufficiently, because of inadequate stomach acid or digestive enzymes, you are left wide open for developing allergies. Your stomach acid (hydrochloric) is the only strong acid in your body. You'll note "acid" in the names of many organic compounds, but these are weak acids.

Eight of the amino acids are essential, that is, your body can't produce them from other amino acids. The essential amino acids are isoleucine, leucine, lysine, methionine, phenylalanine, threonine, tryptophan and valine. Three others— arginine, cystine, and tyrosine—can't always be produced in sufficient quantity by the body. Your body has a mechanism for keeping the proper balance of the essential ones. The amino acids derived from the proteins in your diet mix with "recycled" amino acids in your gut, providing the building blocks (in the proper ratios) for new body proteins. In prolonged fasting or extreme diets, the optimum balance of amino acids can get out of whack, leading to health problems. Both egg and milk have the optimum ratios between essential amino acids and are thus considered to contain the highest grade proteins. Meats are a close second. (Of course, I can't recommend fluid milk until it has been converted to cheese or yogurt.) It is tougher to get balanced protein from vegetables or grains. Thus one must eat combinations of foods in which an essential amino acid rich in one food makes up for the lack of that amino acid in another food. These would be called complementary foods. Corn and beans are a good example of complementarity.

Several amino acids are now becoming important in nutritional therapy for health problems. Thus lysine supplementation helps prevent viruses from multiplying in your body, tryptophan supplementation can help some insomniacs, and glutamine supplementation can help some alcoholics kick the habit. Phenylalanine is found helpful for pain or depression. Tyrosine is being found useful, in conjunction with vitamins, in helping those hooked on cocaine avoid the blues after they quit. The dosages of amino acids used are more than you could ever get from your food.

Carbohydrates are usually divided into two categories: the complex carbohydrates (starches and grains) and the simple ones (sugars). Whole complex carbohydrates are the healthiest. Refined complex carbohydrates, such as white flour or white rice, have retained most of their protein, but have lost most of the other nutrients. Grains and vegetables have adequate protein to sustain life, but fruits do not. (Fruit diets are for the birds!)   Because vegetables are mostly water, one needs to eat large quantities to get significant calories.   On a ratio of nutrients per calorie, called nutrient density, vegetables are the highest of all foods, but vegetable (and grain) proteins don't usually have the best balanced amino acid ratios.

The simple carbohydrates, or sugars, are the extreme in refinement, having lost almost all nutrients.   They even cause a loss of nutrients from your body both while being metabolized and by zapping your sugar regulating mechanisms.   They tend to be quickly digested in the gut, getting into your bloodstream quickly, raising blood glucose levels, and calling forth a strong insulin release.   Oddly, the sugars in some vegetables, especially parsnips but also carrots, tend to get quickly absorbed. If you zap your sugar regulating system for enough years, your body loses its chromium stores and you get symptoms of hypoglycemia. (See Chapter 13.) The symptoms are bizarre— you may find your moods going up and down like a yo-yo. Diabetes can also be triggered in genetically susceptible individuals.

The lipid category of the chemicals of life includes fats, phospholipids, and steroids.   Among fats, there are the fatty acids, which can be saturated or unsaturated.   Animal fats tend to be more saturated than vegetable fats.   Because unsaturated fats are usually liquid, they are also called oils. A saturated fat has all stable bonds along the carbon molecular backbone, whereas the unsaturated fats have from one to four unstable double-bonds along the backbone.   Olive oil is mono-unsaturated, having one double-bond.   Polyunsaturated oils have three or four double-bonds.   The kind of fat you've noticed on your body is a triglyceride, formed by three fatty acids joining to a 3-carbon glycerol molecule.   Triglycerides also circulate in your bloodstream.   Too high a level is considered a risk factor by some, and certainly indicates a metabolic disorder—the origin of which can be nutritional, genetic, or a combination of the two.

Polyunsaturated oils include the only fats/oils that are vitally essential, in the amount of about 1 to 2% of your total food calories. People with dry skin are likely to need extra oils. However, excessive oil consumption requires you to get additional vitamin E to prevent the oils from turning rancid inside your body, which can occur because of the unstable bonds within the oil molecules. The oils are best extracted from the seeds or beans without heat or solvents (i. e., cold-pressed), kept in the refrigerator once opened, and cooked as lightly as possible, if cooked at all.

The essential fatty acids are linoleic acid (found richest in safflower oil), linolenic (in soy oil), and arachidonic acid (in peanut oil). Linoleic acid is supposed to be converted in your body to the other necessary polyunsaturated oils, but it may not happen efficiently in some people as they reach middle age.

Many people are helped considerably by getting some eicosapentaenoic acid (usually abbreviated E P A, or called omega-3 oil). [Rudin '82, Glomset '85] It seems to help keep the blood from clotting too readily, reduces elevated cholesterol or triglycerides, and has many other more subtle benefits. Rich sources are linseed (flaxseed) oil, wheat germ oil, and oils from cold-water fish. This particular oil has been systematically removed from our commercial food supply, for it has the bad habit of turning rancid easily and smelling like fried fish.

The phospholipids have the characteristic of being soluble in the watery matrix on one end of the molecule, but not on the other fatty end. They are found in cell membranes. Lecithin is the best known example of a phospholipid, and is a useful supplement for some people. Two nutrients, choline and inositol, are components of lecithin.

The steroids have a backbone of four interlocking rings and include cholesterol, vitamin D, the adrenal hormones and the sex hormones. Most of the blood cholesterol is produced in the liver and carried through the bloodstream bound to several different proteins. The best known of these are HDL and LDL (high density and low density lipoproteins). HDL is the good guy, and LDL the bad guy. Some extremely vital compounds are made from cholesterol, such as bile acids, which help in the absorption of fats; adrenal hormones, including adrenaline; the sex hormones; precursors of vitamin D; the coverings of nerve fibers; constituents of skin; etc.

With my emphasis on the chemical reactions that take place, I don't want you to picture some sort of a chemical soup. There is a structure and organization to the chemical events, with various levels of organization from clusters of molecules, specialized parts of subcellular units, on up through cells, tissues and organs. View it more as networks of chemical reactions with a different set of reactions taking place in each of the various specialized units. Intermediate reactants are transported both within the cell and through the bloodstream to other parts of the body.

Within the cells are various subcellular units. One type, the mitochondria, specialize in many of the oxidation reactions in which food releases energy. Energy "coinage" is created and stored in the adenosine triphosphate molecule, called ATP for short. ATP will then make its way to another site where the energy is released to drive other chemical reactions. In this process, it loses a phosphate group and becomes adenosine diphosphate (ADP). ADP is then recycled back to ATP.

The cell membranes actively take some molecules in, and refuse entrance to others. Cells are built up into tissues, with the cells cooperating with one another in some mysterious way. The loss of that cooperation is a characteristic of cancer. Each body organ specializes in certain chemical reactions. The liver has been called a biochemical "factory," an apt term if you imagine how factories have to be highly structured and organized to achieve efficient production.

The cells, tissues, and organs live in a very sheltered environment. For example, oxygen must be supplied; carbon dioxide and other waste products carried away; the essential nutrients and intermediate reactants supplied as needed; and a constant temperature and pH factor (acidity) maintained. Water that is lost must be replaced. There are complex mechanisms in your body for regulating the cellular environment. These mechanisms are themselves dependent upon cells and chemical processes, so if the cells that regulate are themselves poorly supplied, the other body cells can't depend upon getting proper regulation. In this manner, parts of your body/mind system can get into vicious circles, with each increasing departure from the norm making it harder and harder to get back to normal.

The circulatory system helps maintain a constant cellular environment. It carries nutrients and intermediate reactants to the cells, and wastes away from the cells, and hormones and prostaglandins that aid in various body regulatory functions to various target organs.

The **heart** is the pump that keeps your circulatory system going. The main fuel of heart muscle cells is fat, whereas other muscle cells mainly run on glucose as a fuel. This modifies the nutrient needs of heart muscle cells slightly, but the cells of your heart are like the other cells of your body in that they need all of the essential nutrients supplied. But the nutrient supply to the heart is far more critical, for the heart never gets a rest. The heart has a higher rate of metabolism than the other organs of your body, resulting in a faster turnover of nutrients, and a greater risk of nutrients being depleted. This may explain why it fails first (and most dramatically) when the nutritional support system lets it down. Animal experiments have shown that the heart may fail with a deficiency of almost any nutrient. In Western countries, the most likely nutrient inadequacies contributing to coronary heart disease are those of vitamins E, B-6 or C, omega-3 oil, magnesium, potassium, selenium, chromium, copper or zinc. Other deficiencies possibly taking part are those of B-complex factors like thiamine, biotin, or trace elements silicon or manganese. Some nutrient excesses that can contribute to heart disease are those of calcium, sodium, iron, cobalt, and vitamin D. You can be born with heart problems if your mother lacked riboflavin, folate, or vitamin A. [Follis '56] Certain non-vitamin nutrients can help in heart disease. One is L-carnitine. [Leibovit '84] Another is pangamic acid.

Because there are individual differences in nutrient needs, different hearts could fail from different nutritional imbalances. But the evidence presented in the next few chapters would suggest that many cases of coronary heart disease in Western countries have a specific combination of nutritional imbalances.

CHAPTER 7

Dietary Drift

Let us look at the drastic changes that have occurred in the American diet since 1860. Some of these changes are implicated in the later emergence of coronary heart disease. Because a number of changes in diet occurred over the same period of time, it is difficult to pinpoint the culprits with the usual type of statistical studies. Thus many past efforts seeking a single cause have led to much confusion and controversy, since there are actually multiple causes.

In 1860, the average American diet, based upon percent of calories, was 12% protein, 25% fat, 53% complex carbohydrates (starches), and 10% simple carbohydrates (sugars). While the changes since 1860 have been gradual, they add up to drastic changes for the century and a quarter. Now the diet is 12-15% protein, 40-45% fat, 22% complex carbohydrates, and 24% simple carbohydrates. [Trowell '81] On average, protein consumption has changed the least, although some individuals may be taking in too much protein. There have been drastic increases in fats and sugars, both of which are nutrient-poor fragments of food. There have been drastic decreases in consumption of nutrient-rich starches, such as potatoes and grains. Furthermore, most of the grains these days have had their germ and bran (fiber) removed.

In effect, many of the most heart-protective nutrients have been stripped from the food supply. These include macro-nutrients like vitamin E, omega-3 oil, magnesium and potassium. Only a fraction of the trace elements found in primitive diets survived. Lost were much of the six trace elements that appear protective of the heart and circulatory system: chromium, selenium, zinc, copper, manganese, and silicon. Some of the major vitamins lost from the basic food supply have been more than replaced by either enrichment or fortification of food. But other micro-nutrients, mostly the more recently discovered ones, were forgotten in the shuffle.

Using U. S. Department of Agriculture (USDA) data in part, let us look particularly at the nutrients-in-the-food-supply trends for this century. [Friend '79, '67; Marston '81] First consider the trends occurring around 1920, when the rate of coronary heart disease was rising fast and first becoming significant. Magnesium, vitamin B-6, vitamin E, and trace element intakes were in a steady downward trend. Increasing steadily at that time were the intakes of fat and milk. Milk became more popular perhaps because pasteurization made milk much safer from bacterial contamination. Milk is a major source of calcium. Vitamin D was discovered and later became popular in the form of cod liver oil. No doubt, the trend toward calcium and vitamin D helped decrease strokes. But all of the trends were adverse to heart health.

Just after World War II, we experienced sharp increases in coronary heart disease. At that time, there were sharply increasing intakes of sodium, calcium, and vitamin D. Total fat consumption was rising steadily. Each of these trends were adverse to heart health.

Coronary heart disease peaked in the 1960's. It is rather curious that two nutrient ratios peaked about that time. These were the dietary ratios of calcium to magnesium, and of sodium to potassium. This could be ascribed to coincidence if it were not for a vast amount of other data, the sum total of which makes a strong case for these ratios being important.

Interestingly, total fat consumption has continued its inexorable rise after coronary heart disease peaked, a fact that helps let total fat off the hook as far as being a direct cause. Saturated animal fat consumption did not increase during this century, so it can not be a major cause.

In the 1960's and 1970's some Americans began taking vitamin pills in earnest. Curiously, the decrease in coronary heart disease since the 1960's matches well to the consumption of vitamin C. [Ginter '79, Verlangieri '85] The idea of a connection is really not so far-fetched, for even mild scurvy tends to promote sudden cardiac death. Note also that the movement toward whole foods and taking vitamins caught on first in California, and that is where heart deaths first started decreasing. [Stallones '80] However, because heart disease rates were decreasing in several other Western countries that didn't experience the vitamin pill-popping fad, it may be that dietary changes were more important than vitamin pills in the earlier phase of the decreases in coronary heart disease.

There is a wide diversity in the diets of the more developed countries, and a wide diversity in the rates of coronary heart disease. Some years ago, several separate groups of researchers noticed that the rate of coronary heart disease in each country went up with the dietary ratio of calcium to magnesium. [Karpannen '78, Varo '74] I have plotted in Figure 1 (next page) the male death rates from coronary heart disease (of males aged 45-74) versus the dietary calcium to magnesium ratio. (Others have plotted the combined male and female death rates.) Also, I've added an estimated data-point for the Masai tribesmen of East Africa. This plot is crucial for sorting out the various dietary factors involved in coronary heart disease.

You'll note that the data points for many of the countries form a reasonable correlation line, although some points are a bit scattered. But the Masai data-point throws matters into confusion. It begins looking more like buckshot hitting a target at random. In scientific studies, a single data-point that doesn't fit one's expectations can yield a valuable clue by forcing a reexamination of all one's thinking.

Therefore, let us look into the Masai life, searching for clues. The Masai are cattle herdsmen. They are apt to drink a few quarts of cow's milk per day, probably half of it fermented into yogurt. Every few days they may feast on a few pounds of beef. This may all be washed down with acacia bark tea. During certain ceremonies, they are known to drink a whole cup of fat. Their intake of cholesterol and saturated fat is the highest in the world, yet the Masai have virtually no

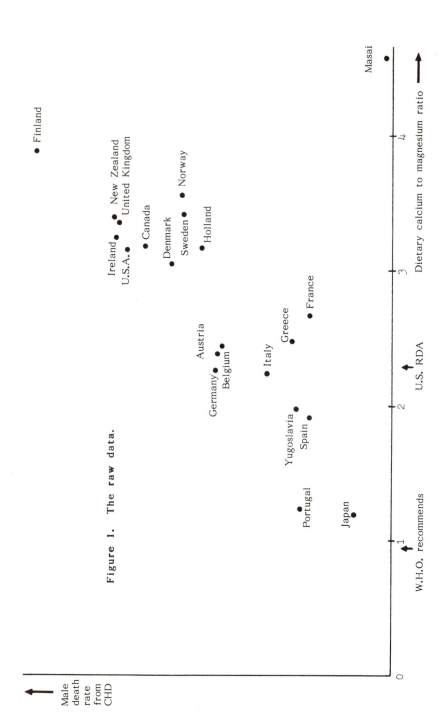

Figure 1. The raw data.

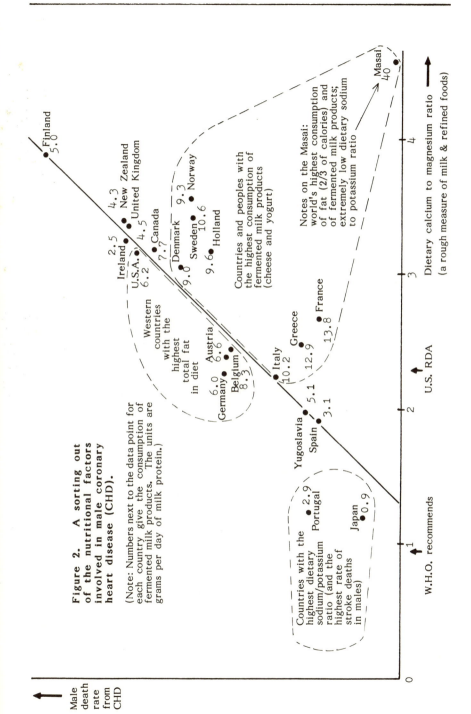

Figure 2. A sorting out of the nutritional factors involved in male coronary heart disease (CHD).

(Note: Numbers next to the data point for each country give the consumption of fermented milk products. The units are grams per day of milk protein.)

Male death rate from CHD

Countries with the highest dietary sodium/potassium ratio (and the highest rate of stroke deaths in males)

Western countries with the highest total fat in diet

Countries and peoples with the highest consumption of fermented milk products (cheese and yogurt)

Notes on the Masai: world's highest consumption of fat (2/3 of calories) and of fermented milk products; extremely low dietary sodium to potassium ratio

Dietary calcium to magnesium ratio (a rough measure of milk & refined foods)

W.H.O. recommends

U.S. RDA

Finland 5.0
New Zealand 4.3
Ireland 2.5
United Kingdom 4.5
U.S.A. 6.2
Canada 7.7
Denmark 9.3
Norway 9.0
Sweden 10.6
Holland 9.6
Germany 6.0
Austria 6.6
Belgium 8.3
Italy 10.2
Greece 12.9
France 13.8
Yugoslavia 5.1
Spain 3.1
Portugal 2.9
Japan 0.9
Masai 40

coronary heart disease and only a minimum of atherosclerotic plaque in old age. The Masai have low blood cholesterol levels, at least those who live in rural areas. There are two protective dietary factors, though. They do not use sodium chloride at all, so that their dietary sodium to potassium ratio is extremely low. They are also the world's greatest partakers of yogurt. Even though the Masai have no coronary heart disease, they do have health problems, such as infections, especially. That may relate more to sanitation than diet. [Biss '71, Day '76, Gibney '80, Ho '71; Mann '72, '64]

Believers in the fat/cholesterol hypothesis of coronary heart disease have mainly chosen to ignore the embarassing Masai data, but some researchers have postulated that the Masai are genetically different from Western man in their handling of dietary fat and cholesterol. It should be noted that the Masai can't be a pure genetic strain, since they have a habit of stealing women (and cattle) from neighboring tribes. Other researchers, grasping at straws, claim that the Masai are protected by a high level of exercise, or by a reduced calorie intake during the dry season.

The data on the Masai could also be an embarassment to believers in the importance of the calcium to magnesium ratio, until we note how some of the countries sort out in Figure 2. Next to the data point for each country I've placed the figures for that country's consumption of fermented milk, which includes both yogurt and cheese. [Seely '81] Notice that increasing consumption of fermented milk products tends to push the data points down and to the right, toward the Masai data-point and toward a lesser rate of coronary heart disease. It appears as if there is a "threshold" level of fermented milk consumption, a level above which there is a significantly lower rate of coronary heart disease. That level would be about 9 to 10 g/day milk protein, or about one cup of yogurt or 1.5 oz. of cheese. If the data-point for Italy appears a bit off, it may be because northern and southern Italians have drastically different diets and rates of coronary heart disease. Thus lumping the Italian data into a single point tends to mislead.

I've circled two countries, Japan and Portugal, which happen to have the world's highest rates of stroke deaths in middle-aged males. [Seely '82] Both countries also have extremely high dietary ratios of sodium to potassium, no doubt from their consumption of salted fish. In contrast, the Masai have the lowest ratio, and all the other Western countries have sodium to potassium ratios in between. It would appear that Japan and Portugal have rates of coronary heart disease somewhat high for their calcium to magnesium ratios, while the Masai rates are on the low side. Therefore, we can conclude that the sodium to potassium ratio is likely to be important in coronary heart disease, as well as in strokes.

Additionally I've circled four Western countries that have the highest consumption of total fat. [Turpeinen '79] They would seem to have slightly elevated rates of coronary heart disease for their calcium to magnesium ratios. But since fat appears to be a weaker determinant of the rate of coronary heart disease than the other factors, there is scant support for the prevailing view of fat as a major cause of coronary heart disease. Further, because high fat diets are generally low nutrient-density diets, the lack of nutrients could be the the more important contributor to heart disease. A low nutrient-density diet could make one's body unable to handle fat properly. (More on this later.)

Now we are left with numerous countries that don't have extremes of fermented milk consumption, of dietary total fat, or of the dietary sodium to potassium ratio. It is appropriate to draw a correlation line through these remaining data-points. We wouldn't try to make the correlation line go through the origin (the "zero-zero" point), for we know that there is an optimum value of the calcium to magnesium ratio different from zero, since both minerals are required in the diet.

The significance of Figure 2 is that the most important dietary associations with coronary heart disease in Western countries are well displayed. The key adverse factors would be high dietary ratios of calcium to magnesium, and of sodium to potassium. An important protective factor would be the consumption of fermented milk products—cheese and yogurt. A minor adverse factor would be total fat consumption. If we had the data from all the world's countries, we would likely find that **all** countries fit into this scheme.

Before ending discussion of Figure 2, we must relate it to the drastic dietary changes of the past century, mentioned early in this chapter. Note that calcium consumption in Western countries is very much a function of the intake of milk and its products; whereas magnesium consumption is very much a function of dietary whole-complex-carbohydrates (whole grains and vegetables). Thus the dietary ratio of calcium to magnesium will go up most in a diet featuring milk and refined foods (refined grains and sugar) with only modest amounts of vegetables. The ratio also depends somewhat on the sources of animal protein in the diet; thus the consumption of red meats raises the ratio slightly, fish lowers it a bit, and fowl has a neutral effect. Obviously, the all-American he-man diet is the worst, containing the least magnesium. But magnesium is not the only protective nutrient found in whole foods. Others are vitamin E, vitamin B-6, trace elements and fiber—mostly lost through refinement. Both fiber and yogurt are apt to be protective by improving intestinal functioning.

At the risk of adding more complexity to the story, I must mention some evidence that gives a new twist to things. From what I've said so far about electrolyte mineral ratios, it would appear that both calcium and sodium are bad actors in the matter of heart attacks. But it turns out that calcium shows a highly protective effect as to high blood pressure and strokes. Thus, the Western countries with the lowest stroke rates take in over 1000 milligrams per day of calcium, and countries with the highest stroke rates take in only about 500 mg/day. Are we then forced to make a choice between having a stroke and having a heart attack? I think not. To see this, we have to consider that in the least developed countries, the calcium intake is certainly no more than 500 mg/day, and that neither high blood pressure nor strokes tend to occur. In these countries, though, the people do not use sodium, and take in generous amounts of potassium from their whole foods. What it suggests to me is that excess sodium, or a high sodium to potassium ratio, causes an increase in the calcium requirements. If those high calcium requirements are met by use of milk, Western peoples are put at risk of heart attacks. However, there appears to be a way out of the apparent dilemma. If you consume whole grains and vegetables, you will have both a low sodium to potassium ratio and a low calcium to magnesium ratio, and should not be at risk of either stroke or heart attack. Those people who are genetically salt-sensitive will probably need to hold down their sodium intake as well.

What is the optimum ratio of calcium to magnesium in the diet? You'll note in Figure 2 that the correlation line strikes the abscissa at a value of calcium to magnesium ratio of 1.3. However, the data do not consider some losses of magnesium during food processing in Western countries (about the same fraction in all). The optimum ratio for individuals may be somewhere in the range of 1.5 to 1.8. Curiously, the World Health Organization (W. H. O.) suggests a calcium to magnesium ratio of about 1.0, whereas the U. S. Recommended Dietary Allowance (RDA) recommends a ratio of 2.3 (calcium 800 and magnesium 350 mg. per day). The W. H. O. figure appears too low, and the U. S. RDA appears too high. Thus it seems that the U. S. RDA has built into it a substantial rate of male heart deaths. But again, it depends upon the intakes of salt and cheese or yogurt.

Research does not have the final answers as yet. Even if a full explanation is not possible at this time, it is clear what dietary changes we have to make. Of importance to commercial interests is the fact that the needed changes don't affect our basic food supply, but only require changes in food processing; that is, milk must be processed more and grains less, and less salt must be added during food processing.

Of interest to women, a graph similar to Figure 2, but using the data on women, shows essentially the same pattern, except more scatter in the data points. More scatter would be expected because the rate of coronary heart disease in women is so much lower than that for men, and there is a greater chance for other factors to be important. In males, the hormone testosterone no doubt contributes to the higher rates of coronary heart disease. Of course, women also have testosterone, but the levels in women are a good bit lower.

Next we will go into more details on the electrolyte minerals and how they relate to coronary heart disease.

CHAPTER 8

More About Minerals

To illustrate some aspects of mineral nutrition vitally important to your health, we'll consider the results of some animal experiments first, and then some human studies.

Nutritional science has relied considerably upon animal experiments during this century. Practically every kind of nutritional deficiency or imbalance has been tried out on animals. The advantages of animal experiments over human experiments are several: they can be more easily controlled, carried out more quickly and less costly, and present fewer ethical problems.

The greatest drawback to animal studies is that the results aren't necessarily applicable to humans. As an example, consider the results of experiments that showed rats have a rather high need for sulfur (from sulfur amino acids, such as methionine, rich in eggs). Based upon that, some researchers concluded that humans have a high need for sulfur. However, once researchers noted where much of the sulfur goes, into making hair, they saw their error. Rats are hairy beasts compared to humans, and need proportionately more sulfur.

There are the often-quoted experiments on rabbits, carried out early in this century. They were fed diets loaded with cholesterol, and developed atherosclerosis. But seldom mentioned are later experiments showing that magnesium supplementation alone will protect the rabbits from developing atherosclerosis when fed cholesterol. [Neal '62] Nor is it often appreciated that in both earlier and later experiments, feeding the rabbits high protein diets from milk protein had an even stronger effect than cholesterol in producing atherosclerosis. [Terpstra '83]

Because rabbits happen to be vegetarian, the results of the unnatural feeding of animal products like cholesterol or milk protein were always of questionable application to humans. Laboratory rats happen to be a much better subject for study, since they are ominvorous like humans. However, rats appear partially protected from heart attacks, possibly because rats produce their own vitamin C. Nevertheless, two separate groups of researchers did manage to produce rat heart attacks. One group did it with a high fat and high cholesterol diet plus an antithyroid medication. Fat was 69% of calories and cholesterol was 5% by weight. [Hartroft '62]

Of greater interest, rat heart attacks were produced much more quickly, effectively and naturally by J. Sós and coworkers in Budapest, Hungary. They used a combination of dietary imbalances alone. For simulating humanlike athero-sclerosis, heart attacks and sudden cardiac death in rats, it was found that the best diet contains excess protein, excess cholesterol, excess salt, excess phosphate, excess vitamin D, and excessively high ratios of calcium to magnesium and sodium to potassium. The diet was 1% cholesterol by weight, 29% protein calories, 21% fat calories, and 50% carbohydrate calories. About 90% of rats died of heart attacks in only five to seven weeks time on the diet. [Sós '65]

Leaving out any one of the adverse dietary factors reduced the rat death rate significantly, but by far the most important adverse factors were the unbalanced electrolyte minerals. Without the high ratios of calcium to magnesium and sodium to potassium, only 13% of rats died. This could be very significant, for you'll recall from the last chapter how these ratios peaked in the American diet about the time that coronary heart disease peaked, and also that these ratios seem to influence the rates of coronary heart disease in different countries.

Of course, the dietary imbalances used on the rats were mostly much greater than would occur with humans. For example, the usual human cholesterol intake is less than 0.1% by weight. Greater imbalances for the rats were necessary to get results in a time span appreciably shorter than the normal rat two-year lifetime. In humans, some factors in coronary heart disease, such as atherosclerosis, may be decades in the making, but a factor like electrolyte imbalance may operate over a modest time span of perhaps months.

The similarities of the rat "heart disease" to the human type were remarkable. Identical blood and tissue changes occurred in the rats as occur in humans. That is, there were increases in blood serum cholesterol, blood pressure, and low density lipoproteins. Atherosclerotic plaques and soft tissue calcifications developed. The rat heart attacks were spontaneous, and were followed by electrocardiographic changes, as found in man. Death tended to occur with recurrent heart attacks. Both blood and heart muscle electrolyte levels changed in the same way as in humans; that is, magnesium and potassium decreased in both blood and heart muscle, and calcium and sodium increased in heart muscle.

Now let us look at the way in which dietary mineral imbalances act in the body—animal or human. The body can tolerate a certain amount of imbalance in the diet without adverse effects, by regulating absorption from the gut, by kidney retention, by fecal excretion, or even by perspiration. Blood serum levels of the electrolyte minerals are fairly carefully regulated, but magnesium appears to be the least well regulated. [Shils '76] The body's normal reaction to stress knocks magnesium out of action. [Altura '80, Flink '79] Magnesium is lost through the kidneys by either alcohol or sugar consumption. Body stores of magnesium can easily get depleted, especially in those on the all-American low-magnesium diet. Because of the importance of magnesium for health, we will be examining the data on it in greater depth. [Cantin '80, Seelig '80, Wacker '80]

One thing we don't learn from all the data we've considered is whether the adverse dietary factors are in milk, or excessive calcium relative to magnesium, or inadequate magnesium, or inadequate vitamins and trace elements which tend to accompany magnesium in food, or possibly all of these. Milk products are the main source of calcium in Western diets. The case of the Masai tribesmen suggests that excess calcium may not be a serious adverse factor, if one gets much of it in the form of yogurt and if one avoids salt. In the human diet, whole grains and vegetables are a main source of magnesium, but these have many more protective factors in them than just magnesium. Vitamin E could be an important one, but trace elements, fiber, and vitamin B-6 could be others. Thus I do not suggest taking just magnesium supplements, for it would be far safer to get magnesium plus all the other protective factors in whole grains and vegetables.

On the surface, some work seemed not to support the idea of the importance of magnesium and the electrolyte mineral ratios. But a deeper examination shows excellent support. For example, hard water was found to be protective in many parts of the world. Magnesium seemed to be the main protective factor. [Anderson '75; Marier '80, '79; Neri '82, '78] But then data from England appeared to prove that magnesium couldn't be the protective factor. [Chipperfield '76] Actually, the English data weren't relevant because there is little magnesium in English drinking water, hard or soft. [Anderson '80] Numerous researchers, misled by the data, came to the erroneous conclusion that magnesium wasn't so important. [Sharrett '79] As a matter of fact, when hard water contains significant magnesium, there is a higher concentration of magnesium in people's heart muscles, and lower death rates from coronary heart disease, with many fewer of the deaths being sudden. [Anderson '75] Water that is hard with magnesium is able to significantly lower the overall dietary calcium to magnesium ratio in localities where the people tend to have a low intake of food magnesium.

In another example, the need appears for a reappraisal of the conclusions reached in another well-known research study. The Irish brothers study compared the rates of heart disease of various sets of brothers. In each set, one had emigrated to the U. S. A. and the other had stayed in Ireland. Those who stayed in Ireland had a much lower rate of heart attacks, got more exercise, ate more whole grains and drank more milk. In Ireland, the dietary ratio of calcium to magnesium turned out to be appreciably lower. [Brown '70] But the authors of the study leaped to the conclusion that it was the exercise that made the difference in heart attack rates, ignoring the possible importance of the whole grains and the lower dietary calcium to magnesium ratio. A recent re-study of the Irish brothers partially corrects the situation, for researchers now find a reduced death rate associated with increased fiber and vegetable intake. [Kushi '85] It appears that the idea of exercise as a protection from coronary heart disease may be fading a bit, and diet is finally getting proper emphasis. (See Chapter 12 for more about exercise.)

Inside the body, magnesium deficiency has numerous adverse effects. It promotes atherosclerosis, spasms of the coronary arteries, blood clots (thrombosis), and loss of magnesium by the heart muscle cells. [Seelig '80, Turlapaty '80, Szelenyi '73] Coronary artery spasms often lead to angina pectoris (chest pains). There is a tendency for heart muscle cells to get selectively depleted of magnesium, while other of the body's muscle cells manage to hang on to their magnesium. [Anderson '75, Behr '73, Chipperfield '78, Elwood '80, Johnson '79, Speich '80] The higher rate of metabolism in heart muscle cells probably contributes to this effect.

Magnesium is really a key electrolyte because it helps to regulate the other electrolyte minerals—calcium, sodium, and potassium. [Burch '79, Ebel '80, Geiderman '79, Shils '76] Magnesium helps keep the "ion pump" in cell membranes working properly, i. e., pumping sodium ions out of the cells, which helps to hold potassium ions in the cells. [Dyckner '81]

The production of energy within the heart muscle cells is dependent upon adequate magnesium. Magnesium is a cofactor for enzymes that produce the biochemical energy stored in the ATP molecule. This energy is ultimately transformed into mechanical work through heart muscle cell contraction and the resultant pumping of blood.

Magnesium also helps maintain normal electrical potentials on the surface of heart muscle cells. [Katholi '79] This is all important for transmission of the electrical impulses that trigger heart muscle cell contraction. An irregular heart beat (called arrhythmia) is a frequent result of magnesium depletion.

A magnesium lack relates to a far more deadly form of

irregular heart beat—ventricular fibrillation, which is a rapid and chaotic contraction of heart muscle cells. [Dyckner '80, Flink '81, Ghani '79, Iseri '75, Loeb '68] Unless interrupted by an electric shock to the chest, or possibly by beating on the chest, death occurs in minutes. Ventricular fibrillation is most likely to happen when there is a sudden change in oxygen supply to the heart, whether up or down. [Lown '79, '77; Verrier '78] Either coronary artery spasms or blood clots could produce the sudden change in oxygen supply. Atherosclerosis could also contribute to ventricular fibrillation by fostering blood platelet aggregation at the sites of plaque (tending to lead to clots) and by worsening the effects of coronary artery spasms (because of narrowed arteries).

The gradual development of atherosclerosis produces a slow decrease in oxygen supply to the heart. This more steady oxygen shortage causes the heart muscle cells to lose magnesium, thus interfering with both the ion pump and energy production. [Polimeni '73] As the situation continues to deteriorate, the heart muscle loses potassium and gains sodium and calcium. At the same time, the normal heart muscle fuel (fatty acids) can't be utilized efficiently, causing further waste of oxygen that is already in short supply. [Opie '80, Janke '75, Lehr '75] At this point, normal everyday stresses could cause damage to the heart muscle cells, and even mild exercise could do it. Because stress itself can cause further magnesium loss, a vicious circle can be set into motion. The result can be self-destruction of part of the heart muscle. This is euphemistically called a coronary event.

In heart muscle cells, the loss of magnesium and potassium, and the gain of sodium and calcium, is a general disorder that occurs in various forms of heart disease, including coronary atherosclerosis, heart enlargement, congestive heart failure, heart attack, and sudden cardiac death. The phenomenon was termed **electrolyte derangement** by W. Raab, who was a leader in biochemical approaches to heart disease. [Raab '69] If the general public has never heard the term used, it is perhaps because events within heart muscle cells haven't received adequate popularization or "PR." The coronary arteries have gotten all the publicity.

In some ways, our language leads us astray in our thinking on coronary heart disease. We use the word "coronary" referring to the coronary arteries, but the problem can be in the heart muscle. We use the word "heart," but the problem may really be a systemic biochemical imbalance of nutritional origin which may lead to atherosclerosis, blood clots, coronary artery spasms, or disruption of the electrical impulses that trigger normal heart muscle contraction. And we use the word "disease," implying an illness, but in actuality it is only a failure of the body's mechanisms for regulation and self-repair, happening because the cells weren't supplied with adequate amounts of the raw materials—the nutrients.

As a research experiment, I obtained from the local coroner samples of hair from middle-aged men who had died of sudden cardiac death. An assay of the hair minerals revealed a unique pattern of levels among the minerals calcium, sodium and potassium. The pattern suggested electrolyte derangement in three out of eight men. Two other men showed toxic levels of lead in the hair, which is often evidence of too low a dietary intake of calcium, magnesium and trace minerals. Thus 62% showed evidence of mineral imbalances being behind sudden cardiac death. (More details in Appendix II.)

Considering all the data, it is apparent that electrolyte derangement has to be recognized as a major factor in coronary heart disease. I have no doubt that it results directly from dietary mineral imbalances, most likely from a low magnesium intake, with possible contributions from other nutrient deficiencies or excesses, from pollutants, or even from bad habits. (We'll examine how bad habits can relate in Chapter 12.)

Next we will look more deeply into the problems with milk in man's diet.

CHAPTER 9

The Sacred Cow

Currently, there is a large and increasing milk surplus. Thus we can expect a new advertising campaign from the milk industry at about the time this book comes out.   The slogan a few years ago was, "Milk has something for everybody."   The answer for some might be, "Yes, trouble!"   The dairy industry should advertise yogurt and cheese more, and lay off pushing milk because of the many health problems it creates.   In fairness, I have to add that the hazards of milk tend to become manifest when there are appreciable refined carbohydrates in the diet.   The combination of these two push you up along the correlation line in Figure 2 (page 41), and become—for men—the deadly duo.

Of all foods, milk produces the most problems.   Among the lesser problems with milk are lactose intolerance, allergies and hypersensitivities.   Lactose intolerance is a genetic trait in which an enzyme that digests milk sugar is missing from the gut.   Milk then brings on diarrhea or other GI complaints. Usually the individuals affected can tolerate small amounts of milk.   Lactose intolerance is experienced by 95% of Orientals; 70% of Blacks; 67% of peoples of Jewish heritage or of Eastern or Central Europe or Mediterranean origins; and 18% of whites in the U. S. A.

Milk allergy can lead to a variety of different symptoms, ranging from subtle to cataclysmic, and usually coming on about a half-hour after ingestion.   If your pulse rate climbs above 85 (normal being about 70) a half-hour after having milk, it is a good clue that you have a milk allergy.

Hypersensitivities to milk can be varied and subtle, and come on hours or days after ingestion. One of the most common symptoms is stuffy sinuses. Even small quantities can get a big reaction. In some men, it is connected to aggressiveness or violence. [McGee '79]

As to milk's connection to coronary heart disease, there is some intriguing evidence:

1. People who have lactose intolerance tend to stay away from milk, and thus have much less coronary heart disease. [Segall '80] This may help explain the generally lower rate of coronary heart disease in American blacks than in American whites. (However, data from the Los Angeles area show more heart disease in blacks than whites.)

2. Men on a milk diet for ulcers have more than twice as many heart attacks on average as ulcer patients on an ordinary diet. [Briggs '60]

3. In Japan, milk consumption went up by a factor of ten over the past 30 years (a far greater change than for any other food). Over the same period, the rate of coronary heart disease went up, and that of strokes went down. Older men seemed to be most affected. [Kimura '83]

4. In Switzerland, a 22% decrease in male coronary heart disease occurred over a 25 year period during which milk consumption decreased 46%. (It is worthy of note that animal fat consumption increased 20% over the same period.) [Guberan '79]

5. In the U. S. A., since the 1960's, there has been a strong movement away from milk, and toward cheese and yogurt. [Stat. Abs. '84] During this period the rate of coronary heart disease has decreased about 30%.

In all statistical correlations, milk is the food most associated with coronary heart disease. [Segall '79, '77] Contrary to the general belief that the problem is in the milk fat (butter or cream), it is more likely in the skim milk fraction (which includes lactose, milk proteins, and various nutrients). According to the work of Stephen Seely, the atherogenic effect of the skim milk fraction is many times greater than that of the milk fat. [Seely '81] The damaging effect is strongest for unfermented milk, with a protective effect seen in fermented milk——cheese or yogurt. Much of the research implicating milk has been published in foreign medical journals.

Research is continuing as to why milk, especially the skim milk fraction, seems to have such an adverse effect. Milk would appear to have a Jekyll and Hyde character: protective when fermented, and damaging when unfermented. (The protective effect of cheese seems amazing, since cheese loses many important protective nutrients in being converted from milk.) The problems with milk could be because of:

1. proteins such as casein or lactalbumin that were found to be atherogenic in animal experiments earlier in this century. [Terpstra '83]

2. lactose (milk sugar) or one of the lactose components, galactose. [Segall '80]

3. lactose promoting lead absorption. [Bushnell '81]

4. the high calcium content of milk, that is, relative to magnesium, as covered in Chapters 7 and 8.

5. calcium absorption being overpromoted by vitamin D fortification. [Kummerow '76, Linden '77, Taylor '80]

6. the pasteurization of milk. [Annand '72] However, even if pasteurization causes problems, the answer is not a return to raw milk with its risks of bacterial contamination.

7. the homogenization of cows' milk, which allows an enzyme, xanthine oxidase, to escape digestion in the gut. The xanthine oxidase then damages arterial walls and heart muscle. [Oster '83, '81, '79]

8. the tendency for phosphorus in milk to bind up the chromium from other foods.

The problems with milk are perhaps a combination of all the above factors. I won't hazard a guess as to which factors are most important. Nevertheless, it is clear what dietary changes we have to make——switch from fluid milk to cheese and yogurt.

Perhaps you have heard of research suggesting that heavy alcohol drinkers and wine drinkers are somewhat protected from coronary heart disease. This could be an incorrect conclusion, for a later study shows that drinkers tend to avoid milk. [Popham '83] There was no significant correlation one way or the other between drinking and coronary heart disease, when the effect of milk consumption was eliminated. This is not to say that alcohol is benign; it leads to nutrient losses. (See Chapter 12.) However, there could be a slight advantage to the evening cocktail, insofar as it acts to relieve stresses built up during the day, and thereby helps protect the heart from stress damage. Milk drinking is more likely connected to coronary heart disease than the drinking of alcohol.

The most popular food guidelines, commonly known as the "Four Food Groups" are biased toward milk (especially the version put out by the National Dairy Council which puts milk up at the top of the list). Also, the U. S. RDA recommends an amount of calcium that could only be obtained through milk products. These guidelines show a gross insensitivity toward the problems that many people have with milk. The W. H. O. is more realistic about matters, appreciating the fact that the less developed countries are not about to develop a dairy industry like ours, especially in view of the prevalence of lactose intolerance. The U. S. RDA for calcium is 800 mg., whereas the W. H. O. recommends 400 to 500 mg.

There has been a strong emphasis in this country on the considerable need of women for calcium to avoid osteoporosis after menopause. Current recommendations of many nutritionists are for an intake of calcium greater than 800 mg. per day. The emphasis should rather be on how to get current levels of dietary calcium into the bones. Absorbed calcium can go astray—it can get laid down in soft tissue, around the joints, on top of atherosclerotic plaque in the arteries, in the kidneys, and in the heart.

The real problem is the body's proper utilization of calcium, and that depends upon many other nutrients. Magnesium is a very important one for helping to get proper control of calcium in the body. [Geiderman '79, Burch '77] The U. S. RDA for magnesium, 350 mg., is set too low for both men and women. Furthermore, many Americans do not even come close to the RDA in their intake, with magnesium intake running 200 to 250 mg. per day. [Schroeder '69, Srivastava '78, Walker '77] The W. H. O. recommendation is far more appropriate: 450 to 500 mg. per day.

Some men don't get enough calcium when they avoid milk

products completely. In societies where calcium intake is low, and sodium intake is high, such as in Japan and Portugal, there tends to be a high rate of strokes. This same situation seems to hold in American Blacks, who get twice as many strokes as whites.

Many of the people who can't tolerate milk can get calcium from cheese or yogurt, or even from old-fashioned heavy cream (excellent in tea or coffee). For those who can't even tolerate these, there are still some excellent alternative sources of calcium. Green leafy vegetables are an excellent source of both calcium and magnesium. From Hispanic culture, there are tortillas and beans. In primitive Mayan areas, the corn for the tortillas is beaten upon a limestone rock, which helps put calcium into the tortillas. From Oriental culture, there is tofu, which is soy bean curd treated with calcium. Another soy product, miso, cannot be recommended as a calcium source, for it is usually too loaded with sodium.

Some additional vegetables that are good sources of calcium and magnesium are cabbage, string beans, carrots, onions and tomatoes. Eggs and peas have adequate calcium. Oranges have good calcium, but it is mainly in the pulp, not in the juice. Meats, unfortunately, contain little calcium and are loaded with phosphorus, which hinders calcium absorption. Soft drinks have similar bad effects.

Primitive man must have sat around the campfire at night and chewed on bones—and no doubt those who grind their teeth in their sleep (bruxism) are trying to do that. Bruxism can often be cured with additional calcium and magnesium. Supplements of bone meal, oyster shell, or egg shell are good sources of calcium. Dolomite contains both calcium and magnesium in a good ratio between the two. There are also various chelated calcium or magnesium supplements, which are usually better absorbed. One should take magnesium as well as calcium, never calcium alone. (Note an exception: People with kidney failure must usually avoid magnesium supplements, following the instructions of the physician.)

Let me mention some useful tips on cheese and yogurt. Many cheeses are 70 to 75% fat calories, and loaded with salt.

Among the worst for salt are Roquefort, parmesan, blue, or the popular processed American cheeses. If you want to watch fat and salt, you might consider using part-skim or low-salt cheeses. Mozzarella is a good example. Note that imitation cheeses are bad news nutritionally. It is uncertain whether or not cottage cheese or buttermilk escape the problems caused by fluid milk.

The idea that yogurt promotes health and longevity is certainly not new. [Douglas '11] The low-fat type is preferred, for the bacterial cultures that make yogurt make less flavorful products from milk fat. Yogurt should contain a live culture, that is, it should not be pasteurized after being cultured. Note that a live culture will get stronger as it ages. Some brands of yogurt may be rich in tyramine, which can produce headaches in some people. In shopping for yogurt, you'll want to check the amount of added sweetener on the label. Plain yogurt, a bit too tart for most American tastes, will have listed about 125 calories per cup and 13 grams carbohydrate per cup. The heavily sweetened form is like a dessert and may have 250 calories per cup and 45 grams carbohydrate per cup. There is a happy medium somewhere in between.

Also, when purchasing yogurt, note that some are more concentrated than others. The watery yogurts may be just right for eating straight from the carton, but may not be as good a buy. You can tell by the protein content per cup—8.5 grams for a typical moist yogurt, or about 12 grams for a concentrated one. The more concentrated yogurt will have proportionately more calories per cup: 210 when plain.

For switching from milk to cheese or yogurt, you'll want to know the calcium equivalents: A cup of milk has roughly the same amount of calcium as a cup of yogurt, i. e., about 290 milligrams. Although cheeses vary considerably in calcium content, it takes about one and a third ounces of cheese to give you the calcium equivalent of a glass of milk.

It is helpful to remember that cows' milk is designed for baby cows—with super high protein and calcium to support the rapid growth rate of a calf—and needs modifying for human consumption.

CHAPTER 10

Controlling Cholesterol

Apparently, two out of three Americans are worried about cholesterol.   But the poll-takers didn't make the important distinction between blood cholesterol levels and dietary cholesterol intake.   If someone asked if you were afraid of the "bogeyman," wouldn't you ask them what they mean by the bogeyman?   I hope to end the confusion and excessive preoccupation over cholesterol with useful knowledge and with ways to bring elevated blood cholesterol levels down to normal. Then no one need worry about dietary cholesterol intake.

Some of the most nutritious foods are rich in cholesterol. It also happens to be a very natural material in our bodies, so it should not be feared.   If you don't eat it, your body will produce it.   Also remember that your body makes many vital substances from cholesterol.

In optimum health, cholesterol production is regulated so that blood serum cholesterol levels run 130 to 150 milligrams per deciliter.   However, with blood cholesterol above about 240 mg/dl, the risk of heart disease is doubled.   Above 300, the risk is tripled.   But then blood cholesterol level is not a good predictor of heart risk, for there are individuals with completely normal cholesterol levels who get heart disease. The connections between blood cholesterol level and coronary heart disease are thus somewhat indirect.

Numerous factors can affect blood cholesterol levels. For example, stress can drastically alter blood cholesterol levels.   An experiment was carried out on a class of medical students: after their "relaxed" blood cholesterol levels were determined, a school exam was announced. New measurements revealed levels more than double. [Pinckney '73]

In less developed countries, blood cholesterol levels run 130 to 150 mg/dl, increasing with age slightly in some cultures, but not in others, and increasing in urban populations as compared to rural populations. The increase in urban environments may relate to increased average stress levels, or it may relate to dietary changes that usually occur when people take up urban life, or to both. [Day '76] The so-called "normal" levels for Americans are set rather high, and expressed in age ranges: 120 to 240 mg/dl for ages 20 to 29; 140 to 270 mg/dl for ages 30 to 39; 150 to 310 mg/dl for ages 40 to 49; and 160 to 330 mg/dl for ages 50 to 59.

The possibilities of lowering blood cholesterol levels by restricting dietary cholesterol are rather limited, with typical effects being blood cholesterol reductions of 5 to 15%. Frequently, the effect only lasts a matter of months, with blood cholesterol returning to the previous levels. This suggests that high blood cholesterol levels are a problem of the body's regulation of it, rather than of excessive dietary intake.

There is somewhat better luck lowering blood cholesterol levels (and stopping atherosclerosis) by going to completely vegetarian diets that are almost totally lacking in cholesterol. For example, 18 out of 39 high-risk males experienced no worsening of their atherosclerosis when put on a vegetaraian diet for two years. [Arntzenius '85] Most likely, such a diet is successful more because it is rich in nutrients and fiber than because it is low in dietary cholesterol. The additional nutrients probably make the body's cholesterol regulating mechanisms work better. With a rather strict diet, Nathan Pritikin drove his blood cholesterol down to 94 mg/dl—an abnormally low level. It was 280 in 1955, before he changed his diet. Upon autopsy, he was found to have beautifully clean arteries. [Hubbard '85] Most likely, there had been a reversal of atherosclerosis. However, I doubt that one needs to go to such dietary extremes to have reasonably clean arteries; the right vitamin/mineral supplements can do as well.

My own blood cholesterol level came out 133 mg/dl at a time when I was eating a diet of nearly 50% fat and including two extra large eggs per day.   I was taking nutrient supplements.   That is the same level as a New Guinea highlander subsisting on an 80% whole complex carbohydrate diet, or a normal male in mainland China, or a Masai warrior in East Africa.   The point I want to make is that people can have widely varying diets of the less refined foods, and can all have ideally normal blood cholesterol levels.   Many Americans may require supplements to get there.

Professionals using nutritional therapy on Americans can generally get the blood cholesterol levels of their patients down to the 130 to 150 mg/dl range, even when the level starts out high.   The nutritional therapist will always attempt to find out in what ways the patient has gotten out of biochemical balance, and try to correct the situation.   There are perhaps twenty different vitamins, minerals, or food factors that can lower blood cholesterol levels.   Different ones will work in different patients, depending upon what ways the patient is out of balance biochemically.   Genetic factors can also be involved.   The nutrients that can be effective are: vitamin A, vitamin C, niacin, vitamin B-6, choline, inositol, pangamate, essential fatty acid (especially omega-3 oil), and the minerals magnesium, calcium, copper, chromium, vanadium, nickel and silicon.   (Refer to Chapter 18 for proper dosages.)   There seems to be a factor in yogurt that lowers blood cholesterol levels.   [Gibney '80, Mann '77]   Other effective food factors are apple pectin, oat bran, and lecithin.

Drug approaches to lowering blood cholesterol levels have been plagued by side effects such as nausea, bloating, gas, or constipation.   Reducing blood cholesterol levels with drugs in men with highly elevated cholesterol levels reduces the chances of a heart attack somewhat, but deaths from accidents and suicides have tended to go up.   [Nutrition Today '84]   Results are better using the biochemical enabling action of nutrients to normalize cholesterol levels, rather than the biochemical blocking actions of drugs.   However, double-blind experiments to find a single nutrient that is highly effective in reducing elevated blood cholesterol levels are more or less doomed to failure, since experimental subjects will vary so widely in their individual nutrient needs.

If you eat no cholesterol, your body will produce the cholesterol equivalent of a half dozen extra large eggs per day. There is nothing wrong with sparing your body the need of making some of that cholesterol by eating a couple eggs per day (if you like eggs, are not allergic to eggs, and haven't already developed serious disorders in cholesterol regulation from unbalanced nutrient intakes). Eggs are better balanced than most foods, being abundant in 30 out of 40 nutrients measured. However, eggs should be balanced with whole grains, vegetables, and fruits.

We need to look at whether dietary cholesterol is fresh (as in eggs, etc.), or has been processed and/or stored. Cholesterol that has been stored for a long time, or has been processed by high heat, forms some breakdown products that are highly effective in producing atherosclerosis. [Kummerow '79, Peng '84] Thus it is best to avoid meat that has been charred in a barbeque, foods deep fried in lard that has been reused, or powdered eggs. (Note that foods deep fried in cholesterol-free polyunsaturates or hydrogenated vegetable oils also contain some hazardous breakdown products. Thus it is best to avoid deep frying altogether.) Fresh cholesterol is certainly the most healthy form, but no doubt you could protect yourself from minor indiscretions by taking vitamin and mineral supplements.

To put cholesterol further into proper perspective, our average diet is only 1 part in a thousand cholesterol. Eggs are about 1 part in 200 cholesterol. Those famous rabbits that developed atherosclerosis were fed one part in 20, certainly a monstrous load for an animal that is vegetarian and lacks the proper mechanisms for handling dietary cholesterol. Recall that supplementation with one single nutrient, magnesium, can prevent cholesterol-fed rabbits from developing atherosclerosis. [Neal '62] Curiously, wolves can handle huge quantities of dietary cholesterol. Man is somewhere in between, adaptable to wide variations in his diet, as long as his foods are not stripped of nutrients.

If your blood cholesterol level is elevated, improve your diet and try supplementing the nutrients that lower blood cholesterol. Then you can stop worrying about cholesterol.

CHAPTER 11

Fear of Fats

The conventional thinking on coronary heart disease has generated a neurotic fear of fats.   Then how come total fat consumption has been rising steadily?   The rise is almost unbroken over the past century and a quarter.   Why haven't you listened to the past generation of "experts"?   If you become frightened by a brush with death, no doubt you will listen, for the nearest expert will point the finger at "artery-clogging fats."

There are two important facts we need to help straighten out the confusion:

1.   We have an innate taste for fat.

2.   Much of food fat is hidden, that is, we don't realize or want to know that it is there.   The food technologists find that processed foods that contain fat sell well——thus they are more than willing to accommodate our tastes.

Relax, though.   **Fat is not inherently bad.**   The problem in a high fat diet is that the fats have displaced other foods of a higher nutrient-density.   Health problems coming from a high fat diet most likely result from the lack of other protective nutrients that help your body handle fats.

We noted in Figure 2 that those Western countries with the highest total fat intake seemed to have an excess of coronary heart disease over and above what one would expect from the dietary calcium to magnesium ratio.   Fat calories were nearly a half of total calories.   But how is it that the Masai, the Samburu, and the Somali tribesmen can get away with diets of about two-thirds fat calories and have virtually no heart disease? If any group of people can get away with such high fat consumption, then fat can not be a direct cause of coronary heart disease. Very likely, high fat is a contributor to coronary heart disease in Western countries because of other nutritional imbalances that disturb fat metabolism. My guess is that the high dietary sodium to potassium ratio is one important imbalance, and another is probably the low dietary magnesium intake common in Western countries. Dietary refined grains and sugars adversely affect both factors.

Another problem of a high fat diet in Western countries is that the fats get modified or have other toxic substances inadvertently added. For maximum commercial profit, animals are caused to grow rapidly by heavy use of grain feeds, hormones, antibiotics or sizable doses of vitamin D. Their flesh is loaded with excess fat through grain feeding, and retains some of the other additives. Excessive vitamin D obtained through the fat and meat supply, combined with vitamin D fortification of various foods and the taking of vitamin D in multivitamin capsules, may overpromote calcium absorption and thereby contribute to atherosclerosis and heart disease. Be aware that the adult RDA for vitamin D is only 200 i.u. per day, and that there may be a long term risk in getting more than five times the RDA, at least for some individuals. [Linden '77; Kummerow '79, '76; Taylor '80]

There is apt to be a hazard in vegetable oils processed in certain ways. [Martin '83] Most oils are extracted using heat and solvents. Heating of unsaturated vegetable oils causes chemical changes, so that some of the molecules will end up in an alien form. Also, the solvents can not be completely removed. Hydrogenation, either partial or complete, produces fats which can not be utilized well by your body's cells. If you insist on eating margarine, at least pick one, such as a tub margarine, that has a maximum of polyunsaturated oils and a minimum of hydrogenation. For myself, I prefer sweet butter and cold-pressed vegetable oils. Note that sweet butter should be stored in the freezer to prevent rancidity. Vegetable oils also turn rancid when stored for long periods of time.

Two oils are hazardous specifically to the male animal:

rapeseed oil and corn oil. [Anderson '78] Rapeseed oil is not commonly used, so is no real worry. With corn oil at 5% of calories, male rats are killed selectively. Since castrated rats are not affected, the action would appear to involve the male hormone testosterone. Since average American corn oil consumption is about 1%, only those few men who get much more than the average may be at risk. In a man, 5% of calories would be about half an ounce of oil per day. In one heart study in which men were fed corn oil, believing the oil to be protective, heart deaths actually increased. [Rose '65]

In Appendix I, I go into more details on the problems of the fat-cholesterol hypothesis of coronary heart disease. The fact that the hypothesis is full of contradictions doesn't seem to slow down its proponents. There is even a certain contradiction in the commercial exploitation of people's worries about heart disease. For example, vegetable oils are heavily pushed as having no saturated fat or cholesterol—but they are 100% total fat!

Researchers supporting the hypothesis, trying to salvage the past few decades of research, have changed the emphasis a bit, focusing more attention on HDL and LDL, both of which carry cholesterol through the bloodstream. The research into lipids may yet yield something of practical value. For example, a precursor to HDL, the apolipoprotein "apoA-I," may become a good predictor of heart risk. That still leaves unanswered the most important question of how to **prevent** heart risks. Apparently, men must worry more than women about HDL and LDL levels for there is an interesting sex difference: at puberty, boys have a significant drop in HDL and an increase in LDL. You can raise HDL (the good one) with supplements of vitamins C and E, by reducing sugar intake, and by increasing exercise. The vitamin C dose needs to be at least 1,000 mg/day. [Bordia '80] Thus you can forget about HDL, LDL, blood cholesterol or triglycerides if you eat more like a primitive man, and also get the right supplements.

For those who are weight conscious, note that fats give you nine Calories per gram, the highest of the three food categories. For comparison, proteins and carbohydrates only give you four Calories per gram.   Thus fats are a concentrated source of caloric energy, and it is easy to overdo them.   It is useful to know that removing 100 Calories per day from your food intake will cause you to lose about one pound per month, assuming that your metabolism is normal.   Of fatty foods, this is represented by one tablespoon of butter, margarine, or mayonnaise.   Two tablespoons of sugar, or 1 oz. of 100 proof liquor, would also have equivalent calories.

To make calorie calculations on food without using food tables, you have to know roughly the water and fiber contents of the foods.   It is handy to know that it takes a much larger portion of vegetables to equal a fatty food in calories, since vegetables have a high water and fiber content.   Be aware that a salad with an oil dressing on it is apt to have most of its calories in fat.   Do not be deceived by regular ground beef advertised as 20% fat by weight, for it actually has two-thirds of its calories in fat.   Many cheeses, including the very popular American process cheeses, are 70 to 75% fat calories. You may not realize the full extent of your fat consumption, since, like sugar and salt, much of it is hidden.   Food manu- facturers know that we have tastes for sugar, salt and fat. They make full use of that fact to get us to buy their products.

Some extremists recommend a diet containing only 10% fat, but most people find that rather unpalatable.   There are also risks in low-fat diets.   [Judd '83]   Problems may occur with absorption of fat soluble vitamins A, D, E and K, and with inadequate essential fatty acids.   According to Dr. Edward Ahrens of Rockefeller University, diets as low as 20% fat can make cell membranes more rigid, blood plasma more viscous, and may reduce immune system function. [Kolata '85]

The average American diet of 40 to 50% fat is likely too much, considering the many modified foods we eat.   There is one health problem that you must consider—high-fat diets tend to promote cancer, especially of the colon and rectum. However, if you get substantial fiber in your diet, especially from whole grains, you will gain some protection.   [Reddy '78]   Supplementation with vitamins A, C and E will confer additional protection.   Thus, if you insist on having a high fat intake, take the necessary steps to protect yourself.

CHAPTER 12

'Bad Habit' Scoreboard

Mostly we've covered good and bad nutritional habits. In this chapter, we'll go into the "bad habits" that are uppermost in the public mind, that is, smoking, drinking, stress/type "A" behavior, lack of exercise, obesity, drugs, etc.

There are important interactions between bad habits and nutritional factors. Knowing them can help you understand better the effects of bad habits. I've used the term synergism before—it is the interaction of two factors to generate an effect far greater than one would expect by adding up the effects of each factor individually. The combined effect can be many times what was expected. One proven example of synergism is the combined effect of smoking and exposure to asbestos dust. The risks of lung cancer are far greater than expected from either risk alone.

This same phenomenon of synergism is highly likely to occur between nutritional imbalances and the so-called bad habits. There is no other way to explain the apparent contradictions pointed out in Chapter 1. Suppose we examine a society in which most of its members share a particular nutritional imbalance. We might find statistically that a particular bad habit carries a high risk with it. However, in examining some other society where that particular nutritional imbalance is rare, we are apt to find that the same bad habit carries a low risk. Thus we can't use statistical methods to determine risk unless we know **all** the important interacting factors. Now you know how, in good faith, "experts" can inadvertently create misinformation!

When the experts say that about half the cases of coronary heart disease can be "accounted for" by conventional risk factors (i. e., bad habits), it does **not** mean that half the cases are "caused by" the risk factors. They are only saying that the possibility of causation exists. With the remarkable correlations found in Figure 2 (page 41), relating coronary heart disease to various nutritional factors, it would seem that there is little room left for considering the bad habits at all. However, we could get caught in the same statistical "trap" as our experts did, if we ignore bad habits while looking at nutritional factors.

A legitimate statistical study of risk factors must include nutritional imbalances as well. That has not been done yet. It is impossible to assess statistically the true risk of the bad habits alone, without taking into account nutritional factors. The true risks will likely be far less than the apparent risks that were figured not taking interactions into account. The epidemiologists need to do a good study comparing the risks of various bad habits in two groups of men: those on the average American diet, and those on a diet which includes whole grains, cheese and yogurt, while not going overboard on salt, fat, sugar and milk. I believe that we have most of the nation indulging in imbalanced nutrition, so that the bad habits appear far worse than they actually are.

Let me cover the most common bad habits in turn: smoking, stress (type "A" behavior), drinking, lack of exercise (or excessive exercise), obesity, drugs, and violent behavior. The tendency to have accidents will also be considered.

Smoking. Among the benefits, smokers say that it helps energize them for work and that it reduces appetite, helping to control weight. I knew one fellow who claimed he couldn't get out of bed until someone put a cigarette in his mouth and lit it for him. The benefits aren't usually appreciated until after the smoker tries quitting.

Among the risks, other than setting fires accidentally, are some very real health problems, such as lung cancer, emphysema, and heart disease. Americans who smoke one pack per day have three times the risk of heart disease, and five times the combined risk of heart disease or cancer. But the validity of these figures is questionable, in view of a likely synergism with nutritional imbalances.

Also, smoking risks may depend upon the way tobacco is grown or treated. Thus, Mexicans get far less lung cancer than Americans, possibly due to the presence of more selenium in Mexican soil and tobacco. Smoking risks may be increased if the tobacco is flue-dried, rather than air-dried.

Curiously, Japanese men are very heavy smokers, but have little coronary heart disease. However, there is a disparity between male and female life expectancies that is nearly as great as that in the U. S. A. Japanese men seem to die of strokes (and other diseases related to high blood pressure) rather than of coronary heart disease. With their many dietary changes of the past few decades, the rate of strokes has been coming down, but the rate of coronary heart disease has been climbing, possibly related to a large increase in milk consumption. [Kimura '83] The Japanese situation appears too complex to be used to give us any clear answers on the safety of smoking.

The data from South Africa are very intriguing. Black South Africans smoke about one-half as much as white South Africans, but have only 1/50 of the rate of coronary heart disease. There are important differences in diet between blacks and whites, with blacks having a diet that is much closer to the primitive ideal or to optimum nutrition. (The same could be said about Mexican diets, that they are more primitive than American diets.) There is a good chance that optimum nutrition could drastically reduce the risks of smoking. No doubt, it is healthiest to have optimum nutrition and avoid smoking—but if you are going to have a bad habit, it is better to smoke than to consume the all-American diet.

Smoking has some very definite effects on your body:

1. It puts small amounts of carbon monoxide and cyanide into your system, robbing you of oxygen. If your vision is getting dim, you may need some vitamin B-12 injections to counteract the bad effects of the cyanide.

2. It puts soot in your lungs, bronchial passages, throat, and sinuses.

3. It tends to stop the action of the cilia (little hairs) that help clear your respiratory passages—exactly the wrong thing to do if you are depositing soot there.

4. The nicotine in smoke produces an adrenaline release, which explains how smoking tends to energize some people. The result is increased heart rate, increased heart output, constriction of blood vessels, increased blood pressure, increased blood serum FFA (free fatty acids), and increased blood-platelet adhesiveness.

The effects of smoking include lower levels of certain vitamins in the blood, particularly of vitamins A and B-6. Vitamin A supplementation will help get the cilia working again. Many nutrients (see list on page 149) reduce blood-platelet adhesiveness, thereby reducing the chances of clots forming in your arteries. Vitamins A, C, and E, and selenium may help protect you from cancer (through their anti-oxidant actions). Vitamins A and C will help your liver detoxify some of the smoking products. Extra B-complex and C vitamins, calcium, magnesium, and some of the trace elements will help you combat the stress on your body resulting from the adrenaline release. Some food factors that may help are pectin, lecithin, alginate, and perhaps others. The worst thing you can do is eat high-calorie, low-nutrient foods.

If you have a smoker's hack, trouble getting your breath, heart disease, precancerous lung changes (or worse), or have been exposed to asbestos dust, it is important to give up smoking, and begin an aggressive program to improve your nutrition. When all health problems disappear, you might be able to take up modest smoking again, but no one will guarantee your health.

Don't think you can escape the risks of cancer by using "smokeless" tobacco (snuff or chewing tobacco). The use of snuff carries a significant risk of cancer of the mouth, in part due to nitrosamines in snuff.

Don't wait for your government to tell you what to do—it acts rather schizophrenic on the subject of smoking tobacco. One part tries to scare the hell out of you to get you to quit smoking, while another part subsidizes the growing of tobacco.

Stress/Type "A" Behavior. We may define stress as the internal reaction to stress-producing events. The way you perceive such events determines the stress you are under. If you do not perceive (consciously or unconsciously) a typical stress-producing situation as threatening, then you do not experience stress. Stress-reduction techniques aim toward changing the mind's way of perceiving events.

The worst sorts of stresses are those conflicts which we have internalized from long exposure, and in which we feel we have no ability to predict or control events. Feelings of frustration, hopelessness and futility can result. Loss of confidence in your ability to cope with your problems is perhaps the ultimate stress.

Our body's mechanism for meeting stress involves the sympathetic nervous system, which gets us ready to meet challenges in which we have to fight or flee. Civilized man's stresses do not generally require actual fighting or fleeing, so that much of the body's reactions to meet stress are not useful. For instance, the adrenaline released because of stress causes your heart muscle to work harder, but because you do not start running or fighting, the energy is wasted.

After a stressful day, there are various ways to turn off your sympathetic nervous system, such as by relaxation techniques, self-hypnosis, meditation, taking a drink, exercise, or other enjoyable pastimes. Repressed anger can be worked out with exercise or punching pillows, which is far better than punching your boss or taking it out on your family.

In type "A" behavior, stress feeds upon itself and becomes reinforced over and over. The sympathetic nervous system is activated much of the time. The individual may not realize that he is in a constant state of stress. Symptoms of type "A" behavior are irritability, overactivity, intense drive, sense of urgency, hostility, inability to relax, worrying and insomnia. Of these, hostility is perhaps the most significant. [Friedman '84, '82, '80]

Curiously, a number of stress symptoms are similar to those of magnesium depletion. I suppose we could have a "which came first?—the chicken or the egg?" argument over stress and magnesium depletion. The fact is, stress depletes you of magnesium; and magnesium depletion enhances the bad effects of stress. [Gunther '80] Magnesium would seem to have a key role in keeping the body from overreacting to stresses. The mechanism is likely to be as follows: when under stress, the adrenaline that is released causes free fatty acids (FFA) to be poured out into the bloodstream. The FFAs can yield the energy necessary for fighting or fleeing, but FFAs also tend to bind up magnesium, taking it out of action. [Flink '79, Turlapaty '80] If body magnesium stores are low, the central nervous system has a tendency to become over-stimulated. [Chutkow '80] With the mind keeping the body mobilized for action, further magnesium is lost. Under these internally generated stresses, the body has a tendency to use up many different nutrients faster than the diet can possibly supply them. With the brain constantly stimulating the heart, and the heart's nutritional support system inadequate, the heart is likely to sustain damage after prolonged stress. Thus a vicious circle occurs, which can ultimately lead to a heart attack. The health breakdowns from stress are most likely to happen in the heart, the immune system or in the stomach. [Beamish '85]

Nutritional therapy can have an important role in preventing stress damage. Practically all nutrient needs are increased during stress. Vitamin C may be the most important nutrient lost during stress, but magnesium runs a close second. The all-American low-magnesium diet helps to make stress an important risk factor in coronary heart disease.

It would be interesting to speculate that part of the American knack for getting things done depends upon being slightly depleted of magnesium. But some individuals go too far. With poor dietary habits and under heavy stress much of the time, they may become seriously depleted of magnesium and set themselves up for a heart attack. With optimum nutrition and good vitamin and mineral supplementation, stress should not be a risk factor at all.

Drinking. The effect of drinking on your health depends upon how much you drink, how long you've been doing it, and how you "dry out." A drink after a hard day's work is probably beneficial, helping you unwind and forget the cares of the day. That old story about losing a certain number of brain cells with each drink is an improper extrapolation from animal experiments. True, you will lose brain cells with heavy drinking, especially at older ages, and especially if you neglect your nutrition.

Heavy drinking appears to be an important cause of death in males aged 45 to 65. Long-term heavy drinking leads to cirrhosis, a liver disease which may come on without warning. It can happen in a few years of drinking or in a lifetime. Alcohol is metabolized in the liver, and excess amounts tend to pickle the liver. If you've already had some adverse liver changes, your drinking days are over (assuming you wish to avoid a helluva way of dying).

Those who tend to have weekend drinking bouts are exposed to a special risk. The cessation of drinking puts a heavy stress on the body the day after. This was found out in dogs who were induced to drink. A few dogs experienced heart attacks during the withdrawal phase. In men, strokes tend to increase the day after drinking cessation. Also, sudden heart attacks occur more often on Monday than any other day of the week. [Rabkin '80] The combination of the stress of drinking cessation plus the stress of going back to work on Monday perhaps contributes to the excess Monday heart attacks. But recall that stress damage may result partly from nutrient depletions, as noted in the last section. Those who taper off their drinking with a "morning eye opener" or "some of the hair of the dog that bit them" may be reducing the stress of drinking cessation. However, they also need some good nutrition, as you will see.

There are some very important nutrient losses noted in heavy drinkers. Among the nutrients that are known to be lost are vitamins A, C, E, B-1, B-6, B-12, niacin, folate and the minerals calcium, magnesium and zinc. (Iron may appear to be lost, according to blood measurements, but it tends to accumulate in the liver.) No doubt many other nutrients are lost as well, so that complete nutritional therapy for heavy drinkers would be a wise move.

Alcohol is addictive, and many who decide to quit will

have difficulties quitting. Involved in alcohol addiction are genetic and psychological factors, as well as nutritional-biochemical factors. But before you decide to take up "religion" or long term psychotherapy to help you quit, note that there is an amino acid supplement, glutamine, that can help many quit, without side effects. See the book, "The Prevention of Alcoholism Through Nutrition," by Roger J. Williams (Bantam 1981). Note that it takes much more glutamine to do the job than you could ever get from food. It takes about 2 grams of glutamine per day (500 mg. doses at each meal and at bedtime). Glutamine can be obtained from your local health food store or from mail-order vitamin companies.

One thing about alcohol, it seems to increase confidence, while reducing judgment and capabilities. Thus, while under the influence, you must avoid operating cars, boats, airplanes, guns—or other deadly weapons.

Lack of exercise/Excessive exercise. Exercise has been a bit too heavily promoted as a protection against heart disease. The statistical association of less coronary heart disease among those who get moderate exercise does not prove that exercise protects. After all, there can be factors that lead to coronary heart disease that also make a person less desirous of partaking in exercise. I have no doubt that there are such factors, and I'll bet they are nutritional.

Skeptical thoughts about the benefits of exercise are raised by data from eastern Finland, where there is a high rate of heart attacks among loggers. They would certainly seem to be prime physical specimens, leading an active life outdoors. Curiously, the soil in eastern Finland is somewhat depleted of magnesium, and thus both food and drinking water contain less than the normal amount of this element. [Holtmeier '80]

Also casting doubt on the exercise hypothesis are the number of experienced marathoners, appearing in excellent health, who keel over dead suddenly. Even Jim Fixx, the guru of running, went out that way. In fact, the rate of sudden cardiac death among runners is about seven times that of non-runners. [Thompson '82] No doubt this only applies to Western countries. Consider the Australian Aborigines or the

Tarahumara Indians of Mexico, who do considerable running and also live on primitive diets. [Connor '78] Sudden cardiac death or other forms of heart disease are unknown in these peoples (until tribal members take up "civilized" diets).

In our society, we have a tendency to confuse fitness with health. No amount of physical training can guarantee you a healthy heart. You can appear to be (and feel) physically fit, but you might still be on the verge of a heart attack. Optimum nutrition gives you the best chance of having a healthy heart. In fact, if you are not getting good nutrition, it is best to avoid heavy exercise.

Moderate exercise does have some benefits—it increases HDL, the good lipoprotein in the blood. Exercise helps keep calcium in your bones. It also helps burn off calories that might otherwise go into fat. One advantage of a nutritional therapy program is that it will make you feel more like exercising. You don't have to have a grim look on your face when you are working out—you can actually enjoy it.

If you are an athlete, you would want a diet that is the modern equivalent of the diet of the ancient Olympic athletes (see Chapter 5), featuring many whole complex-carbohydrates with modest amounts of meat. Experiments have shown that athletes have the greatest endurance on such a diet. Extra amounts of certain nutrients may aid performance: vitamins C, E, and the B-complex; minerals zinc and selenium; and the non-vitamin nutrients pangamate and L-carnitine. [Leibovitz '84]

Carbohydrate loading is a technique useful in athletic events where you have to put forth maximum energy for more than a couple hours. Starting nearly a week before the event, you would avoid training, eat a high-protein/low-carbohydrate diet for a few days, then load up on carbohydrates for the next few days before the race. This puts more glycogen stores into your system. Some say this technique is dangerous, leading to heart arrhythmia, but that is unlikely if you tend to eat whole foods year round.

Some athletes take anabolic steroids to help build up muscle for competitive sports. This causes some hormonal imbalances, with reduced sperm production. There is some attendant risk of liver cancer or heart disease. After quitting steroids, male breasts will enlarge for awhile, until body hormones achieve balance again. Perhaps nutritional therapy could help protect an athlete using steroids.

You should be aware of certain physiological effects of exercise on your body. Exercise causes release of endorphins, which are sort of a natural "morphine." Thus exercise is likely to make you feel better. The danger is that exercise can easily be overdone, resulting in injuries. Also, note that excess exercise, such as running more than 40 miles per week, has been shown to lower testosterone levels and sex drive.

Obesity. The standard line is that obesity results from too high a caloric intake relative to the exercise level. That is quite true, but other problems could be present. First of all, the metabolism may have gone awry, so that the individual is unable to burn fuel fast enough. Secondly, the appetite mechanism may not be functioning well. Since these problems are at the cellular level, there is a reasonable chance that getting all the essential nutrients to the cells may correct the problems.

You should forget about all those heavily advertised "crash" diets. They will foul up your metabolism in such a way that you will actually **gain** weight in the long run. The only effective long-term diet is moderate calorie restriction, especially of foods that have many calories and few nutrients, such as sugar, fat and alcohol. Add to this an increased exercise level, plus vitamin and mineral supplements.

Drugs. This vast topic could be a book in itself. There are many ways of categorizing drugs: as legal or illegal, prescription or over-the-counter, socially acceptable or not, addictive or not, stimulants or tranquillizers (uppers or downers), safe or dangerous, psychoactive or not, etc.

Alcohol, coffee and tea have to be included as drugs. Note that the caffeine in coffee or tea can have some benefits, if you don't overdo it. It can give you temporary additional mental or physical energy, or relief from allergy symptoms. But three cups per day of coffee can cause a significant loss of nutrients from your body.

An important aspect of drugs is that they tend to have anti-nutrient effects. [Roe '84] Thus, aspirin will deplete you of vitamin C and folic acid. Barbiturates, used in some sleeping pills and tranquillizers, will interfere with vitamin D metabolism. Diuretics will knock out B-complex and C vitamins, plus calcium, magnesium, potassium and zinc. Digitalis tends to knock out vitamin B-1, magnesium and potassium. The list is almost endless.

Mainly, I want to cover helpful ways of getting off addictive drugs without suffering the torments of the damned. Nutritional therapies can be helpful, but have been little publicized.

The body builds up tolerance to increasing doses of many drugs. In fact, the desired effects from the drugs require ever increasing dosages—but then there is hell to pay getting off them. Some common withdrawal symptoms are headaches, anxiety, nervousness, tremors, palpitations, sweating, cramps, energy loss or drowsiness. Psychotic reactions can occur.

The best news is that vitamin C in large doses can be immensely helpful when you are trying to quit an addictive drug cold-turkey. However, in order to avoid bloating your belly with large doses, it must be a non-acidic form of vitamin C, such as calcium ascorbate or sodium ascorbate. Oral dosages of 1 to 2 grams **per hour** are considered reasonable for kicking heavy drugs like heroin. If you can find a knowledgeable physician or clinic that helps people quit, you can get vitamin C intravenously. Kicking milder drugs like coffee may require only a few grams per day of vitamin C.

Some clinics use both niacin and vitamin C, especially if there are psychotic reactions to either the drug or its withdrawal. Dosages of both vitamin C and niacin might run 3 to 5 grams per day of each. The vitamin C dose should not be less than the niacin dose. The niacin dose must be worked up to gradually and should not exceed 3 to 5 grams per day. Niacin is not a do-it-yourself nutrient in these large doses. A physician must perform periodic liver function tests.

The usual approach to kicking a heroin habit has involved use of methadone. Many who have gone this route have said that methadone is harder to kick than heroin. Oddly, heroin is not addictive for those who need it to control pain. In England, terminal cancer patients are given heroin cocktails daily, and they are able to be pain-free and lead relatively normal lives up to the end. If the cancer regresses spontaneously, the patient has no trouble going off the heroin.

Cocaine enjoyed great popularity in the 1890's. Even Sigmund Freud was promoting its use, until after he saw some of the bad effects. Performance may be enhanced with initial or rare use, but will deteriorate with regular use (according to many recent sports figures who've gotten deeply into it). There is a high death rate associated with cocaine use. The overstimulation of cocaine is believed to lead to circulatory collapse. I suspect that a poor nutritional state adds to vulnerability. Coronary artery spasms and a heart attack can occur, even with clean arteries. [Schachne '84] Currently there are some research efforts to help people kick cocaine more comfortably. The withdrawal blues can be reduced using vitamins with the amino acid tyrosine.

I'll bet that the urge to do drugs, the risks of addiction and the risks of a bad trip are all increased when an individual is in a poor nutritional state. When it comes to psychoactive chemicals, I prefer highs from modest amounts of coffee, mocha or English-type tea. (These stimulants helped me write this book.) Protected with some vitamins and minerals, I am able to keep a real tiger in my tank.

Violence. No doubt we've all had the urge to do violence at one time or another, but factors like self-control or ethical considerations have stopped us. Much of violence takes place within the family and is unreported. Those who can't or won't keep the lid on their urge to do violence can end up in jail. It is men, far more than women, who get into trouble with violence or crime—mostly young single men.

A wide range of factors may contribute to violence. Psychosocial factors are of great importance. However, underlying nutritional imbalances could contribute to adverse psychological factors, such as reduced self-control, hyperexcitability, irritability, mental instability, negative outlook, antisocial feelings, difficulty in relating to other people, sudden rages, or even psychotic behavior. (See next chapter.)

How do we interpret the fact that the consumption of several foods—meat, milk or sugar—correlates statistically to violence? Meat seems to increase aggressiveness in men, but that will only contribute to violence when an individual is already at the edge of it. Milk may contribute to hyperexcitability through its high calcium to magnesium ratio, or by triggering a cerebral allergy. [McGee '79] Typical amounts of sugar consumption in the U. S. A. can lead (over a long period of time) to hypoglycemia, which is a fertile source of antisocial behavior. It was found that 90% of the men in one jail were hypoglycemic. By shifting diets toward foods of higher nutrient-density (avoiding sugars, excessive fat, and food additives), various juvenile detention facilities have experienced substantial decreases in antisocial behavior among inmates. [Schoenthaler '85, Schauss '80]

Some other factors may be important. An excess of copper can lead to a proneness to violence. Accumulation of toxic metals like lead may contribute to hyperexcitability and violence in some individuals. Alcohol and drug habits have been suggested as causing much violence. However, the more fundamental problem may be the poor nutritional state of people on alcohol, on drugs, or with accumulated lead. Recall that alcohol and drugs tend to deplete a person of many different nutrients. It has also been found that alcoholics tend to be hypoglycemic.

It would be a mistake to try to ascribe any "main causes" to violence. There are a variety of contributing factors that interact and develop over a long period of time (possibly a lifetime). A poor diet may act like a trigger. A long-term poor diet could destroy an individual's chances of bettering his life. Thus, in an adverse social milieu, he might find that the easiest path to take is one leading to crime and violence.

Accidents: Mostly we've heard about a slow reaction time making people accident prone. But, also contributing to accidents are any factors that reduce your awareness of what is happening around you. When your brain is functioning at its peak, there are many "channels" by which important sensory information can reach your consciousness. However, if you are in a poor nutritional state, doing drugs or alcohol, in a powerful emotional state or overly fatigued, you will be more susceptible to having an accident. I wish to mention a few nutritional and non-nutritional factors that may be important.

Hypoglycemia could put you into a state of mind where you become accident prone. If you are deficient in zinc and/or copper, you may get a tendency to "space out" a bit. That can contribute to an accident. If you are in a marginal nutritional state relative to zinc, switching to a vegetarian diet (normally healthy) could give you a "spacy" feeling.

A non-nutritional factor is the concentration of charged ions in the air you are breathing. Some people are more susceptible than others to problems from the depletion of negative air ions. The modern design of our cities, our buildings and our cars have a tendency to knock out negative air ions. Places where you'll find a rich supply of negative ions are at the seashore with onshore breezes, next to water-falls, in the shower and in the woods on a breezy day. If such places make you feel a lot better, you might also want to try out a negative ion generator in your home, office or car.

If the air is well charged with negative ions, you are apt to feel good, but if charged with positive ions (or none) then accident rates go up and heart attacks are more frequent. A fascinating book on the subject is, "The Ion Effect," by Fred Soyka (Dutton '77/Bantam '78).

*   *   *

I hope this chapter helps you better understand some of your bad habits, so that you can either enjoy them more safely or break their hold upon you more easily. Remember that the bad habit you must give up is less-than-optimum nutrition. Optimum nutrition will help reduce the ill effects of the other bad habits. As a side effect of optimum nutrition, you may also find that it helps break your addiction to a bad habit.

(A caution for women planning to have children: Nowhere more than in pregnancy are the benefits of optimum nutrition proved, and the risks of bad habits like smoking, drinking and drugs demonstrated. No doubt, interactions of nutrition and bad habits are important. But still, the unborn child must be given the benefit of any doubts.)

CHAPTER 13

Keeping Your Head Straight

When people are hurting in the mind, they are apt to pay a high price to anyone who offers hope of relief.   Of all pains, psychic pain may be the most difficult to bear.   Rather than running to a psychotherapist first, one's best strategy might be to see a nutritional therapist.   If the root of the problem is inadequate nutrition, no amount of psychotherapy will cure it. Even if the primary root of the problem is in the psychologic realm, nutritional therapy can probably help shorten the period of psychotherapy needed.   Whatever, nutritional therapy will not be all that time-consuming or expensive.

There was a time when the medical community denied the importance of nutrition to brain functioning.   At one time, Western philosophers were able to consider the mind and body as separate.   No longer is that possible.

Your mental well-being depends upon genetic, nutritional and environmental factors.   Additionally, the attitudes you choose to take toward your life situation are extremely important.   Thus it looks as if there is free will.   You are not a mechanistic robot unless you fail, or are unable, to use the higher centers of your brain.   That can happen when there has been poor psychic integration from too many internal conflicts, or when nutrition has been inadequate.

Even with free will, there is a chemical basis to your thought processes, the same as with other body processes.   A less than optimum nutrition can adversely influence brain chemistry, and therefore interfere with normal thought processes.   [Hoffer '83]   As an example, consider the case of psychological depression. Studies have related depression to marginal deficiencies of vitamins B-1, B-2, B-6, B-12 or C, where depression was measured by objective psychological tests. Deficiencies of, or an extra need for, any one of these vitamins can cause depression. The shocker is that psychological symptoms almost always develop before any physical symptoms of the deficiency. [Brin '80]

The balance of nutrients is crucial to normal mental functioning. By shifting nutritional balances, some deranged minds can be made whole and some normal people can become a bit crazy. The susceptibility to mental problems from nutritional imbalances varies widely among individuals. Nutritional therapy, usually called megavitamin therapy or orthomolecular psychiatry when applied to mental derangements, can help tranquillize the overwrought man or stimulate the lethargic man. More subtly, finding your own optimum nutrition can help make your brain/mind work better. It can give you more brain power, heighten awareness, make you feel better, and make you more able to cope with stress.

Many mental problems have been approached successfully by supplementing with one or another nutrient, or a combination of nutrients. Unfortunately, a nutrient that works in one case won't necessarily work in others. Identical symptoms may require different nutrients. In other words, individual differences are all-important. Double-blind experiments to determine efficacy are often useless, primarily because of the nearly impossible problem of finding "matched" controls, that is, persons with similar genetics and in a similar nutritional state. Thus the individual best serves as his own control, with the nutrient alternately given and taken away.

Consider some examples of nutrients that have been found to work in individual cases:

1. If you are a burn-out case, and have lost all your ambition, you might find a dramatic restoration of ambition by taking a few hundred milligrams per day of pantothenic acid.

2. If you are primarily involved in intellectual work, you may find that zinc and copper supplementation sharpens up your brain, allowing better creative imagination.

3. If you do physical work, you may find that iron

supplementation gives you more energy to get the job done.

4. If you are a lethargic type of person, you may find that copper or bioflavonoids energize you.

5. If you are hyperactive (usually a male problem), driving everyone around you crazy, you may find that you have excess copper, or toxic levels of lead, or are getting too little magnesium for the amount of calcium, or have a food allergy.

6. If you are anxious much of the time or have insomnia, you may need more magnesium.   Other cases of insomnia could be helped by GTF-chromium or by the amino acid tryptophan.

7. If you are irritable or have a bad temper, you might find great help from magnesium or GTF-chromium.

8. If your memory has been failing in recent years, you might need extra zinc and vitamin B-6 (especially if you have white spots on your fingernails), or magnesium, or choline.

9. If you need tranquillizing, you might find the answer in magnesium, zinc, inositol, vitamin C or vitamin E.   On the other hand, if you take a prescription drug to calm yourself, you may become addicted to it.

10. If you get depressed too often, you might find relief with magnesium, GTF-chromium, or B-complex and C vitamins.

Experimentation is necessary to find out what answers your own personal needs.   Psychosocial factors need to be considered.   Also, any of the problems mentioned above could have its roots in a food allergy.

Hypoglycemia: To be strictly correct, this should be called functional or relative hypoglycemia.   It actually means that blood sugar is unstable, and drops low at times.   Because of the many possible mental symptoms, we'll consider the topic in this chapter, even though there are many physical aspects to it as well.   Among the mental signs are depression, insomnia, being chronically anxious, constantly irritable, having crying spells, various phobias, inability to concentrate, forgetfulness, confusion, unsocial or antisocial behavior, chronic restlessness, psychotic episodes or suicidal urges.

Some physical symptoms that may go with hypoglycemia are: chronic fatigue, chronic nervous exhaustion, a need to eat often to avoid hunger pains or faintness, faintness if meals are delayed, fatigue that is relieved by eating, getting shaky when hungry, getting sleepy after meals, or getting sleepy during the day.   If you have a number of these symptoms or signs, then you may be suffering from hypoglycemia.

The supplement that helps hypoglycemics the most is GTF-chromium.   Also helpful are general vitamin and mineral supplementation, having a high-protein breakfast, avoiding liquids at mealtime, going easy on fruit, avoiding refined carbohydrates (sugar and white flour) and eating frequent small meals.   Many have to avoid foods high on the glycemic index, which is a useful ranking of foods as to how hard they zap the blood-sugar regulating system.   [Crapo '84, Jenkins '84]   High-protein diets can be used as a temporary measure, along with vitamin/mineral supplementation.   However, I feel that the primary importance of a high-protein diet is to slow down digestion, so that the sugar regulatory system doesn't get zapped so hard.   For the long term, you must restore chromium levels and correct any other biochemical imbalances.

Contributing to hypoglycemia can be such factors as chronic stress, lack of exercise, weak functioning of the adrenal glands, insufficient stomach acid or allergy.

The usual medical test for hypoglycemia is the glucose tolerance test (GTT).   You are given a cup of water with a half cup of sugar dissolved in it, on an empty stomach, and then your blood sugar levels are measured for the following six hours.   During the test, it is worthwhile to write down how you feel at various intervals.   It is necessary to write it down at the time, since you likely to have a memory blackout.   If you are hypoglycemic, you are likely to experience some of the following: trembling, cold sweats, headache, dizziness, rapid heartbeat, numbness, irritability or blurred vision.   The more symptoms you have, the more likely you are hypoglycemic.

The interpretation of the results of the glucose tolerance test seems to depend upon who is doing it.   The test may be brutal and unnecessary in many cases.   Also, blood sugar levels don't necessarily relate well to the mental symptoms.   Perhaps symptoms come from rapidly changing blood sugar levels that disturb the balance of brain neurotransmitter chemicals.

Hair mineral analysis offers a useful alternative to the glucose tolerance test for hypoglycemia. Sufferers usually have a hair chromium level that is at least three times below the normal level. The lower the hair chromium level, the more likely that the person has problems in blood sugar regulation.

While hypoglycemia can make you feel as if you are going crazy, you really aren't. Let us now consider the small percentage of people (1 to 2%) who really are mentally ill. Psychiatrists put various labels on them like schizophrenic, manic depressive, etc. The labels may not be all that meaningful, for I know of one psychiatric institute where all the labels on the patients changed when the institute got a new director.

The causes of mental illness can be looked at in various ways. There is definitely a genetic predisposition to it, but it is generally triggered by the environment. Drugs can control it, but tend to make "vegetables" of those treated. A better approach would be high doses of the right nutrients; nutritional therapy can help many lead normal lives. Controlled experiments have shown better results for megavitamin therapy, as compared to conventional treatment with drugs. With megavitamin therapy, a lower percentage of patients had to be readmitted to the hospital, and those readmitted required fewer days in the hospital.

A number of researchers have been working at developing more meaningful categories for classifying the mentally ill, based upon biochemical differences noted in mental patients. [Pfeiffer '75, Watson '72] Carl C. Pfeiffer, Ph. D., M. D., divides schizophrenics into the following groups:

1. nearly half of schizophrenic patients need large doses of niacin, vitamin C, vitamin B-12 and folate;

2. one out of six needs calcium, zinc, manganese, lithium, methionine, thyroid hormone and antidepressants, but must avoid folate;

3. about a quarter need zinc and vitamin B-6; and

4. most of the remainder have a cerebral allergy or have an allergy to wheat gluten.

An important fact to be noted is that the treatment of the first group of schizophrenics requires a totally different set of nutrients than the second group, and that treating the second group with nutrients used for the first group will make the second group worse. Thus a single megavitamin program (such as the one featuring niacin and vitamin C) for all schizophrenics will show only modest overall improvements— with one group improved and another group made worse. This could explain some poor results in the early days of megavitamin therapy, so often quoted by its opponents. (Those who practice conventional psychotherapy seem to have considerable antipathy toward the practice of megavitamin therapy.)

In more recent research, EPA or omega-3 oil (from linseed oil) has shown striking benefits for some cases of schizophrenia or of neurosis. [Rudin '82]

There are also megavitamin treatments for some forms of senility, and for a variety of childhood behavioral disorders. These latter come with "labels" such as retarded, slow learner, minimal brain dysfunction, dyslexia, hyperactive or autistic. The labels tell us next to nothing about the underlying nutritional biochemical disorders. Sometimes testing reveals toxic levels of lead or cadmium to be behind the childhood problems. [Maugh '78, Pihl '77]

In covering this subject, I mostly want to show that there is hope for many of the so-called mentally ill. I want to emphasize that megavitamin therapy is not a do-it-yourself enterprise. It requires a megavitamin therapist, orthomolecular psychiatrist, or an M. D. of the nutritional specialty.

I'll end this unfinished topic with a speculation. I sometimes get the feeling that the flowering of both science and psychiatry during this century are related somehow to the dietary drift covered in Chapter 7. Nutrition has improved in many respects, but the emergence of a variety of nutritional imbalances could be driving some of us a bit crazy, fostering creativity in others through hyperactivity or abnormal competitiveness, and causing many to flame-out in their prime.

CHAPTER 14

Sex and Nutrition

(Because this chapter is written from a male point of view, some women may not wish to read it. However, it has much useful information for women.)

If Mother Nature's goal is to multiply our species, then it seems that she has programmed men rather well in the matter of sex. Messages with sexual overtones have a direct hotline into the male brain, interrupting all other incoming data.

With all the constant titillation by subliminal advertising (when you buy the car, the beauty comes with it), by "T and A" on TV, sexy-looking playmates in the magazines, adult movies, etc., it's a wonder we ever get any work done. We need to gain insight into our biologically-programmed male sexual urges in order to achieve some detachment and peace of mind. We would probably overpopulate the world worse than it is, if it were not for our cleverness at birth control.

We are in a youth-oriented culture, but we obviously can't maintain youth forever. To maintain our attractiveness to the opposite sex, we have to stave off the ravages of time. If you allow yourself to become fat, toothless and flatulent as you age, you will have to scale down your expectations. Also unattractive are a paunch, bags under the eyes, heavy body odors, prostate problems, heavy snoring, and being too tired much of the time. If you have frequent illnesses or other infirmities, you'll have to find a woman who is looking for someone to mother. If you develop hemorrhoids, you'll find them decidedly inconvenient when you are having sex, for, as you get excited, your hemorrhoids will get excited too.

Having to take heart or high blood pressure medicine, or having to worry about getting too excited, is a real turn-off to a woman. While men may joke that the best way to depart from this world is just after a great orgasm, remember that no woman wants to live with the guilt of having contributed to your flame-out by heart attack.

In some ways men are luckier than women. We are fortunate that women don't judge us on good looks as often as we do them. Also, as we age, we seem to have more women from which to choose.

Many of the problems that interfere with your sexual attractiveness can be prevented, or even reversed, with optimum nutrition and nutritional therapy. No matter how far gone you are now, it is worth an effort. It will help you feel better about yourself and help keep a mate from deciding that you are over the hill.

One thing that is very important, if you have a good mate now, you should work together with her, both of you working toward optimum nutrition. You don't want to get too far ahead of her or else she'll start feeling insecure, believing some other woman is going to steal you away.

The male hormone testosterone is certainly a key to male sex drive. Super-aggressive males perhaps have too much of it being produced and floating around their system. Those who are very passive and have minimal sex drive may be underproducing. If you are a regular marijuana smoker or a heavy drinker, you may find that your testosterone levels are low. Something else that lowers sex drive is the food preservative, nitrate (always rumored to be added to the food at Boy Scout camp to keep the boys from getting horny).

There are some nutrients that seem to influence sexual capabilities. They aren't likely to fulfill male fantasies of superhuman sexual feats, but they certainly can bring males up to normal—which is sexy enough. It is doubtful that young males need anything, although optimum nutrition raises the possibility of first-rate sexual performance without a dragged-out or spacy feeling the next day. You see, when you indulge heavily in sex, you use up nutrients and other biochemical compounds (enzymes) that are needed for other physical and mental functions.

One of the more important nutrients used up in sex is zinc. Each male orgasm causes the loss of one to two milligrams of zinc. That may require 5-10 milligrams in the diet to replace because zinc absorption in the gut is far below 100%. If you don't replace the zinc, you'll gradually deplete your body stores. Then, as you age, you may get a variety of ailments, including poorer intellectual functioning and prostate problems. Tiny white spots on your fingernails are one sure sign of zinc depletion.

While on the subject of zinc, I must warn you about some interactions of zinc with other trace elements. Prolonged zinc supplementation may interfere with the body's level of copper, manganese, selenium and iron. I know one fellow who had been taking about 50 milligrams daily of zinc for a year, but no copper, and developed the rather peculiar ailment of painful spasms in his penis after orgasm. The problem disappeared after he added a 3 mg. copper supplement to his regimen and reduced the zinc to 30 mg. In general, the ratio of zinc to copper in a supplement ought to be about 10 to 1. It is much more likely for a man's copper level to become too low than too high. The reverse is true of women. Men who are hyperactive, or get all their water through copper plumbing, should probably avoid copper supplementation.

One biochemical compound involved in sexual abandon is histamine. Its release leads to a blushing reaction and the warm feeling before orgasm. Those who are slow in or have difficulty achieving orgasm (men or women) may need extra chemical precursors to histamine. The B-complex factor, folic acid, is an important one. In the U. S. A., B-complex tablets are limited to 0.4 milligrams of folic acid, to help assist doctors in identifying cases of pernicious anemia. If you use a high dose tablet of the other B-complex factors, you may end up with an imbalance, shorted on folic acid. Many will find benefit in taking a couple folic acid tablets with their B-complex tablets. Don't let it bother you that the strongest folic acid tablets available over the counter, 0.8 milligrams, say that they are for pregnant or lactating women. (In Canada, 25 mg. folic acid tablets are available over the counter.)

Another nutrient that is a precursor to histamine is the B-complex factor, niacin. Niacin is likely to get a response in 10 minutes, whereas the folic acid response happens in a matter of days and seems more natural. Even modest doses of niacin lead to a rapid flush reaction in most people, which is why B-complex tablets usually contain another form of the vitamin, niacinamide, which gets a slower response. You have to experiment to see what works best for you, but don't go overboard on any one nutrient, since that can create imbalances that disturb other biochemical functions.

While the problem of being unable to get an erection may have psychological roots, it can also be physiological. It is generally worth trying nutritional therapy first, since that can help reduce time needed for psychotherapy later. A gradual degeneration of the circulatory system with aging can be behind the loss of the ability to get an erection. That can be reversed partially by nutritional therapy.

Now let us look into what can be done to improve your sexual attractiveness. Nutritional therapy, tailored to the individual, can frequently do wonders, but may take many months of time to work. I'll cover the specific nutrients or other factors that can help in many of the problems. (Note: For the appropriate nutrient dosages, see especially Chapter 18.)

Obesity: As pointed out in Chapter 12, the important steps to weight reduction are cutting down on calorie intake, switching to foods of higher nutrient density, increasing exercise, and fixing up a faulty appetite mechanism (or faulty metabolism) by using vitamin and mineral supplements. Also, sex is excellent exercise. In other words, take your mate rather than a plate.

Having a paunch: Although genetic factors are apt to be important, you can improve matters by exercising the belly muscles. For keeping your connective tissues from failing and letting your innards sag, the most important nutrients are vitamins C and B-6, copper and silicon. The same applies to sagging jowls and neck wattles.

Bags under the eyes: This is a sign of excess fluid in the tissues. However, if you have dark circles around the eyes, it tends to suggest allergies, or else too little sleep. To drive fluid out of the tissues, the most important nutrients are vitamins C and B-6, and magnesium. For tightening up skin, try vitamins C and B-6, copper and silicon. Nutritional therapy can do almost as well as a face lift but may require a year's time to notice a difference.

Rotten teeth: No one ever seems to mention the fact that in the skeletons of primitive people, only a few percent of teeth are found decayed or missing. And all that primitive people had were twigs or bone slivers to use as toothpicks— no toothbrush, toothpaste, or dentists. Your teeth depend for their health upon the quality of your saliva and the health of your gums. If your teeth happen to be somewhat loose, it may mean that you are losing calcium from your jawbone. Sugar is considered the number-one enemy of teeth, and fluoride the ultimate benefactor. Unfortunately, there is a total neglect of many other nutrients that are also important for maintaining the health of your teeth. Chief among these are vitamin C, vitamin B-6, bioflavonoids, calcium, magnesium, phosphorus, molybdenum and strontium. If you eat too many refined foods, fluoride treatment could actually contribute to other health problems. Nutrients in excess that may promote tooth rot are selenium, copper and/or vitamin B-1. Selenium would only be a problem in certain parts of the midwest where the soil is loaded with it. Bad breath is brought on by many of the same factors that lead to tooth problems.

Flatulence: This means excessive gas, either trapped and causing you pain or released with social embarassment. Too many legumes (dry beans, soy beans or lentils) or improperly prepared legumes can do it. You may need yogurt and more food fiber regularly to keep the right bacteria working in your lower intestine. Food allergies also cause gas. Or you may be producing too little stomach acid or pancreatic juices, which can often be fixed up with nutritional therapy.

Heavy body odors: Deficiencies of either magnesium or zinc can contribute to excessive odors.   Deodorants and antiperspirants work partly by blocking your skin pores.   They don't get at the real, biochemical problem.

Heavy snoring: If your snoring is as loud as a 747 taking off, or a jackhammer at 10 feet, you probably have a health problem (and your mate has a sleeping problem).   I know that there are some nutrients that help, for I was a heavy snorer before trying vitamins and minerals but a fairly light one afterwards.

Excessive Fatigue: Among the many possible causes of fatigue are allergy, nutrient deficiencies, poor thyroid function, anemia, or exhaustion of the adrenal glands.   Proper thyroid function requires adequate amounts of certain trace elements such as iodine, zinc, manganese, nickel and bromine. Anemia can result from a variety of nutrient deficiencies (or extra needs) such as of iron, copper, nickel, folic acid, vitamin B-12, pantothenic acid and other B-complex factors.   For those who tend to get fatigue in the afternoon, it has been found that a high-protein breakfast helps.   Numerous tests and trials may be required to determine the cause of fatigue.

Hair loss with aging: Heredity appears to be one of the more important factors here, but it is possible to slow down the loss with optimum nutrition.   The shortage of (or extra need for) almost any nutrient can contribute to premature hair loss, but zinc and high quality protein are perhaps the most important factors.   After trying vitamins and minerals for a few months, some people find a profuse number of new hairs growing just outside the hairline.   Receding of the hairline appears to slow down as long as the supplements are continued.
    A drug originally developed by Upjohn Company for high blood pressure, minoxidil, happens to restore recently-lost hair in some men when applied externally in a salve.   [Olsen '85]
    As to greying hair, some have claimed that supplements of brewer's yeast, pantothenic acid or PABA have restored color.   However, these nutrients have only worked on a small

proportion of people. The use of hair-darkening agents containing lead is not wise, since the lead is absorbed and finds its way into the bloodstream and bones. [Marzulli '78]

Prostate problems: Usually these involve enlargement, bacterial infection or cancer. The bladder is pushed aside by the enlarged prostate, so that bladder capacity becomes very much reduced, and one has to get up during the night to urinate. Zinc is the most protective nutrient for the prostate gland, but essential fatty acids, vitamin E, vitamin A and vitamin B-6 help get zinc back into the gland. Many men have had prostate enlargement disappear using these supplements, and thus have avoided the surgical knife. It takes a year to get the results, and unfortunately, it doesn't seem to work with all men. Prevention is best. Note that prostate problems don't seem to exist in the less developed countries.

Hemorrhoids: Essentially, these are varicose veins of the anus. From the commercials with the evening TV news, you may gather that there is big money in preparations to relieve hemorrhoid symptoms. You can bet that they don't advertise in the less developed countries, since hemorrhoids don't tend to exist there. About one out of three Americans suffer from hemorrhoids. While stress can make latent hemorrhoids act up, it is certainly not the cause. The problem is one of nutrition and is cured by getting extra fiber, vitamins A, C, E and B-6, essential fatty acids and bioflavonoids. The fiber helps bring the fecal cylinder up to normal size (larger) so that the evacuation mechanisms can work easily without straining at stool. You should increase fiber gradually, to avoid getting a blockage. The nutrients help restore the structures and restart the glands that produce the lubricants that aid stool passage. Once you get your defecation equipment working right, you'll find that you spend only a minute on the throne, that it is a pleasant experience, and that there is little or no soilage around the anus.

Frequent illnesses: If you get illnesses more than a few times per year, you might want to tune up your immune system.

(However, families who have recently entered young children in school can expect additional illnesses.) Optimum nutrition can strengthen your immune system. The immune system needs all the essential nutrients for proper functioning, but the nutrients that appear most important are folic acid, zinc, and vitamins B-6, B-12 and C. Also helpful are bioflavonoids and pangamate. Vitamin A seems to help you resist bacterial infections. Lysine can help resist viral attacks. (Limit daily dosage to 1.5 grams.) Note that stress can make your immune system work less well, but with optimum nutrition, stress may be unimportant. Too many polyunsaturated oils in your diet, or high doses of vitamin E (1000 i.u.) can also impair normal immune system functioning. For those whose immune systems are hypersensitive, i. e., they get allergies, a high dose of vitamin E and less dietary protein may be the answer. Identifying allergies and eliminating the problem substances will give your immune system a better chance of fighting off the real enemies (bacteria and viruses).

When your body is responding to infection with a fever, supplementation may not be wise. Thus you should fortify your system while you are well.

Herpes: If you have the genital herpes virus, you may wish to join one of the herpes support groups. The virus is supposedly only passed on when you have an active herpes sore. But still, many potential partners wouldn't want to take the chance. Some sufferers may be helped by vitamin C or by the amino acid lysine. Lysine appears to inhibit virus multiplication, whereas another amino acid, arginine, seems to foster virus multiplication. Since nuts, peanuts and chocolate are rich in arginine, the herpes sufferer might want to avoid them. High doses of BHT (butylated hydroxytoluene, a preservative) are claimed to help. Some drugs are being tested, but they only seem to help on the first appearance of herpes. Optimum nutrition plus tuning up your immune system (see above) should help reduce the problem.

Infertility: While many couples are trying to avoid having [more] children, there are also quite a few trying to have children and can't.   An infertility problem can be either in the male or the female, or partly in each.   Whatever, nutritional therapy of both partners can improve chances.   Sometimes the male sperm count is too low.   In that case, there are several possibilities to check out:

1.   If you've been wearing a jockstrap or jockey-type undershorts, it may be keeping your testicles at too high a temperature.   Optimum temperature for healthy sperm production is about 70° F.   The higher the temperature above that, the greater the fraction of defective sperm you'll be producing.

2.   You have probably accumulated some P C B (polychlorinated biphenyl), which tends to reduce sperm count.   It is a common environmental pollutant, for 90% of Americans have accumulated detectable levels in their fatty tissues. Vitamins A and C can help combat this problem.

3.   General nutritional therapy may help.   The nutrients most critically necessary for sperm production (DNA synthesis) are adequate protein, zinc, folic acid and vitamins B-6 and B-12.   Vitamin E will increase sperm count in the man and decrease chances of a miscarriage in the woman.

Excess fertility: If you already have all the children you want, you might want to consider a vasectomy, which is a 20-minute office procedure.   About 14 million men have had a vasectomy.   Some earlier work on monkeys suggested that vasectomy increased the chances of atherosclerosis, but later research suggests no detriments to human male health.   Some possible problems: About 1% of men get inflammation of a sperm-collecting duct.   Also, about 60% of men develop antibodies to their own sperm, but that doesn't appear to create any significant problems.

Acne: There are a variety of causes.   For many, the two most important nutrients for combatting acne turn out to be zinc and vitamin A.   Others may be helped by avoiding iodine, in either seafood, iodized salt, or in vitamin and mineral supplements.   Food allergy is another cause of acne.

Stuttering: This is mostly a male problem. It is not all that common but it can cause a man to withdraw socially. Some cases, at least, can be helped by sizable doses of vitamin B-1 in the order of 50 mg per day. An important co-factor required for vitamin B-1 to work properly is magnesium.

Gout: This is another mostly male problem, occurring especially in hard-driving men. Huge doses of folic acid, about 80 mg. per day (unobtainable in the U. S. A.), can usually cure the problem. Other nutrients can also be important: A copper lack can contribute. Excesses of polyunsaturated oils at the level of 15% of calories can elevate uric acid levels, worsening gout. Rich foods must be avoided, as your doctor will tell you.

Backache: This isn't very convenient for making love and other activities. It may have its origins in muscle imbalance, back injuries, or nutritional or psychosomatic factors. Psychological factors usually build upon other minor physical problems with the back. In fact, when you can stop your frustrations and other psycho-social problems from creating tension in your back muscles, most of you will be well on your way to cure. Tension in the back muscles interferes with blood circulation to the back area, leading to back pain or muscle spasms, or even to shooting pains down a leg. Special exercises can help many, especially exercises that relax back muscle tensions, and strengthen both back and belly muscles. Helpful to some are vitamin C in multi-gram doses or general nutritional therapy. Before allowing surgery for a back problem, it is best to exhaust all other possibilities. For a second opinion, you might read the book, "Mind Over Back Pain," by Dr. John Sarno (Morrow 1984).

High blood pressure: If you are taking a beta-blocking drug, and it is causing impotence, get your doctor to consider something else. (Caution: Do not go off the drug without your physician's approval.) You may want to go looking for an M. D. of the nutritional specialty who might cure you of high blood pressure (or heart disease).

High blood pressure deserves considerable attention for it is so prevalent in the developed countries and so rare in many of the underdeveloped countries. Now, I'm not talking about those blood pressure peaks you may get either during sexual abandon or by diving into cold water (peaking about 300 mm Hg). It is when high blood pressure is prolonged for many years that it can lead to heart disease, stroke, kidney failure or blindness. It is very much related to nutrition, and the best approach to the problem is through nutritional therapy. Mostly you hear about excessive salt consumption being the cause of high blood pressure, but there are actually many possible causes. If you have it, you must identify the factors that are most important in your particular case. Possibly you'll need the help of a nutritional therapist to sort out the many possible factors.

The possible causes or contributors to high blood pressure are: obesity; excess alcohol consumption; excess sodium intake (in genetically susceptible individuals); excess chloride intake; excess intake of nitrates; deficient intakes of calcium, magnesium, potassium, copper, zinc, vitamin A or vitamin C; inadequate intake of unsaturated fat or excess of saturated fat relative to unsaturated; exposure to cadmium or lead; exposure to pesticides; and/or allergy. [Kaplan '85] Garlic can help in some cases. Biofeedback or relaxation therapy may help reduce blood pressure slightly.

Certainly, as a first approach to the problem, you might try eating more like primitive man.

*   *   *

Of course, you don't need to get rid of these health problems just for sexual reasons. You'll find a greater overall enjoyment of life in many ways.

CHAPTER 15

Assorted Hazards

Hardly a day goes by that the newspapers or TV aren't exposing a new environmental hazard—pollution of our air, food, drinking water, workplace, or even our homes, with toxic metals, pesticide residues, defoliants, herbicides, solvents and other exotic chemicals. If we listened to all the "experts" on the hazards around us, we might end up a quivering mass of jelly. What then is our best strategy?

Some may try to forget it all; some may develop neurotic worries; and others may join protest groups and lobby for changes. But there is an excellent way of protecting ourselves that we don't hear much about. It is by stimulating our own body's natural defenses with optimum nutrition and with certain supplements.

Hundreds of millions of years ago, man's animal ancestors evolved defenses against toxic substances. We needed these defenses, for some of our common vegetable foods contain mild toxins. Most likely, plant toxins evolved to protect the plants against insects. If we eat a variety of foods, our livers won't get overloaded with any one food toxin. Nowadays we have to contend with many man-made hazards. We must avoid the worst of the hazards around us, and then quit worrying about the rest of them. Efforts to rate the various hazards is continuing within the scientific community. [Ames '84, '79; Calabrese '81, '80]

Among the hazards are the **free radicals** produced in our bodies by low-level radiation, toxins, rancid oils and even as a side effect of normal metabolic processes. These energetic fragments of molecules create havoc by attacking the structures of the body's cells and interfering in normal biochemical processes. The anti-oxidant nutrients—vitamins A, C, and E and the mineral selenium—work at destroying free radicals before they can do damage. Free radicals may be involved in the initial arterial damage that leads to atherosclerosis. Other possible damages are breaks in our genetic material, which are a first step on the path to cancer. Amazingly, our bodies happen to have a defense, using special enzymes which repair breaks in the strands of our genetic material.

We must keep the rate of repair going faster than the rate of damage from all the factors that tear down our bodies. Damage is usually reversible in the early stages but becomes irreversible when it has gone on too long.

There are considerable individual differences in the response to environmental pollutants. Some individuals are hypersensitive, getting symptoms right away. Could they be the lucky ones, forced to avoid the irritants—while others of us might continue exposure and later get cancer?

Many exotic chemicals have been introduced into the environment since about 1950. They are very unfriendly to living things. There is bitter irony in a company slogan like "better living through chemistry." Cleaning up the environment will take a lot of time and money, and things are likely to get worse before they get better. In California, there is progress, for officers of some companies breaking pollution laws now go to jail.

During this century, several thousand different food additives have been introduced into the food supply, at least into processed foods, and it is impossible to know how safe they are. However, we can not condemn all of them. There are preservatives such as BHA and BHT that actually appear beneficial. Another type of preservative, nitrates or nitrites, can be bad news; but its worst attribute, that of being converted to cancer-causing nitrosamines, can be prevented with vitamin C.

Some of our hazards are side effects of the revolution in agriculture. Excess nitrogen fertilizer tends to enter the water table, and pollute our water supplies. Pesticides kill the 99% of beneficial or innocuous insects to knock out the one percent of insect pests. Pesticides also kill earthworms that aerate soil, thereby inhibiting beneficial soil bacteria from working. Pesticides persist long enough to pollute our water supplies and concentrate as they go up the food chain. Pesticide residues kill birds and are a subtle hazard to us as well. As for myself, when I find insect tracks in my celery or worm tracks in my apple, I almost feel relieved to know that the food is able to support life. We must all discipline our senses to prefer an inconsequential visible blemish to a hazard that is large and unseen.

When people first crowded into cities, disease and pestilence thrived with the increased problems of sanitation. Human wastes got into well waters and disease epidemics became commonplace. The engineers developed safer water supplies and sewage disposal. But all these systems are compromises which tend to sacrifice some earlier benefits. For example, water treatment removes nutritional minerals from the water, frequently adding toxic aluminum or excess amounts of sodium. The water is softened, making good wash water, but not the healthiest drinking water.

Exotic chemicals and solvents have found their way into the water table in many parts of the country. Water supplies that use river waters have another problem: humus in the water reacts with chlorine, forming carcinogens. Also, the older water supply pipes tend to add lead to the water, especially if the water is acidic. The pipes in our modern homes will add copper, beneficial to some individuals but bad for others. Plastic pipes will add cadmium, toxic to all. The water is usually so wretched tasting that many have taken to typically non-nutritious beverages.

A good spring water is perhaps healthiest. Those collecting and storing their own spring water need to know that the jugs must be stored in the dark to avoid algae growth. Jugs that are to be reused must sometimes be washed out with baking soda to prevent the water from getting a moldy taste. The fact is, a good spring water supports all kinds of living things—including yourself.

No matter where you work, you are likely to be exposed

to some pollutants. With more tightly sealed offices or homes, to save energy, you now get more exposure to gases slowly coming out of the building materials. One is radon gas, which gives you an unexpected radiation exposure. Others could be solvents coming from glues, or formaldehyde coming out of foam insulation or from cabinets made of pressed wood. Or you might become allergic to various synthetic materials. Also, in a fire, the smoke from burning plastics can do you in.

Your employer has a duty to inform you of any hazards from the things you work with and to provide protection. The trouble is, your employer isn't likely to know anything about stimulating your own body's defenses. Thus, if you work with solvents, you should know that they will dissolve the natural oils from your skin or from cells inside your lungs. Additional oils in your diet can replace the oils lost from your skin only very slowly. A wheat germ oil lotion on the skin can help to minimize the damage. Mineral oil lotions may be worse than nothing. Solvents are also absorbed through the skin and will raise havoc with your innards. If your liver doesn't detoxify them fast enough, the liver itself can get pickled.

For general protection against environmental pollutants, wherever they are found, you can take supplements of vitamins A, C and E. The appropriate dosages for most people are in the range of 10,000 to 25,000 i. u. of vitamin A, 1,000 to 4,000 mg of vitamin C, and 100 to 400 i. u. of vitamin E. Note that the U. S. RDAs take no account of the extra need for nutrients because of environmental pollutants. You've probably heard "experts" warning you against vitamin A dosage at these levels, but they never seem to tell you that vitamin E will protect you from vitamin A overdosage. Note well that once you've been on supplementation of vitamins C and E for awhile, you should not abruptly quit supplementation, for that will bring on deficiency symptoms. If you plan to quit, then taper off the dosage over several months' time.

We are all being exposed to **toxic metals,** some more so than others. Those who work in or live near a smeltering plant get the most. Some toxic metals have been around for thousands of years, but their levels have increased drastically in more recent times. However, the Romans may have been done in partly by lead used in pewter plates and cups. In dealing with the toxic metals—lead, aluminum, cadmium, mercury and arsenic—fortifying your own body's defenses is all-important. A hair mineral analysis is useful for finding out your body load of toxic metals. (See Appendix II.)

Lead: There are a number of nutrients that will help prevent lead absorption or help clear it from the body. It is most important to get adequate amounts of the minerals calcium, magnesium, zinc, iron and selenium. Vitamins C and E are important. Methionine, an essential amino acid that is rich in eggs, helps clear lead. [Mahaffey '80, Singh '79] Lactose (milk sugar) promotes lead absorption. [Bushnell '81]

There is a lot of lead dust on the ground, especially near busy roads, because of tetraethyl lead in gasoline. It has been noted that short dogs accumulate more lead than tall dogs. The same must hold for children, especially growing ones, who would be laying down lead in their bones.

Lead is a real problem for adults, too. Using hair mineral analysis, I found high levels of lead in the hair of two out of eight men who had died of sudden cardiac death. I've also found high hair-lead in numerous men with health problems. Frequently, it relates to inadequate intakes of calcium, magnesium and trace elements. However, in some cases, it wasn't significant, for they had used hair-darkening agents containing lead acetate. That is not wise, for the lead is slowly absorbed and finds its way into the bones. [Marzulli '78]

Aluminum: A generous magnesium intake does the best job of blocking aluminum absorption. Phosphate and fluoride also work against the absorption of the 50 mg. or so of aluminum that goes through your gut every day. Antacids that contain aluminum hydroxide are best avoided. Some drinking water supplies contain aluminum, left over from the precipitation of suspended matter with aluminum compounds. It is not wise to cook or store acidic foods (citrus, tomato, cherry or rhubarb) or oxalate foods (spinach, other greens) in aluminum pots. Otherwise, aluminum cooking pots are fine. Aluminum is not usually a problem in your body unless it manages to get through protective barriers that keep it out of the brain. In the brain, it leads to an early and irreversible senility.

Cadmium: When cadmium is absorbed by your body, it tends to accumulate in the outer layers of the kidney and lead to high blood pressure. The symptoms depend upon the level of exposure, with extended low-level exposure leading to kidney damage and high blood pressure, and heavier exposures leading to more usual symptoms of toxicity. The "Ouch Ouch" disease in Japan was from cadmium. Some sources of cadmium are tobacco smoke, zinc smelting plants, and the torch-cutting of old galvanized tanks. You can help your body block cadmium absorption by getting adequate zinc and selenium. Some other nutrients that also help are calcium, copper, iron and vitamin C. [Pfeiffer '78, Venugopal '78]

Mercury: Mercury compounds can poison the brain. At one time, mercury was used in making hats; and the most heavily-exposed workers became known as "mad-hatters." Modern sources are some fungicides used on grain seeds, or eating fish from waters downstream of industrial plants that make paper pulp or chlorine. Dentists are much at risk from breathing in mercury vapors while making mercury fillings. About 1% of people are hypersensitive, and can't take mercury fillings in the mouth. Selenium supplementation is the best way of preventing problems with mercury.

Arsenic: A little bit of arsenic is good for you; in fact, it is an essential nutrient. However, too much will do you in. The British used it to knock off Napoleon. Getting adequate selenium is the best protection from excessive arsenic.

* * *

In summary, your best strategy against the various environmental hazards is to:

1. Mobilize your own body's natural defenses with optimum nutrition and the specific supplements that help.

2. Avoid the worst of the hazards around you.

3. Then quit worrying.

CHAPTER 16

Enjoyment of Food

Want to know how to make people mad? Just try to tell them what foods they should be eating! This illustrates how culturally loaded the subject of nutrition is. Thus it is best for me to approach the subject cautiously.

We have to keep in mind that foods are for enjoyment as well as for nutrition and health. Every culture develops its own food habits, and these habits evolve with time. Those cultures that maintain a strong tradition of nutritious foods and eating habits can flourish for the longest time with their peoples in the best health. However, in the U. S. A., we seem to be developing a melting-pot cuisine of foods that are smooth, require a minimum of chewing, and can be bolted down fast. The foods are devoid of fiber and loaded with sugar, salt and fat. When combined with two major staples like refined flour and milk, the result is a high rate of male heart disease.

In Chapter 5, I suggested that we are led astray by innate tastes and have to acquire self-discipline. To see the truth of this, consider a few examples:

First, as children, we are admonished to stay out of the cookie jar and not to eat too much candy or ice cream. Thus we learn discipline early but we don't learn the reasons for it. Later we have to be told to watch our liquor. If we revolt against this discipline during adolescence, we are apt to develop habits that will lead us into trouble.

Second, we've heard what happens to people when they first get exposed to these "goodies" as adults. American Indians went crazy over alcohol when first introduced to it.

Also, Eskimos went wild over our sugar-bombs. Of course, their tribal elders saw the dangers and told their peoples to stick to the old ways. But how many listened?

Finally, throughout history, there have been movements towards whole foods, but the message always gets forgotten or distorted with time. [Robinson '77] If there were no innate tastes leading man astray, the message would have stuck and been incorporated into the culture.

In ancient times, Hippocrates, the father of medicine, was apparently stressing the importance of healthy food. Around 400 B. C. he was recommending whole grains, vegetables and fruits. Obviously, the message didn't stick or we would have physicians everywhere recommending these foods. In recent times, Denis Burkitt, M. D., has been one of the more vocal medical advocates of healthy food. Over a half century before him was Sir Robert McCarrison, M. D., all but forgotten. You may read his paper, "Faulty Food in Relation to Gastro-Intestinal Disorder," in the Journal of the American Medical Association for January 7, 1922, pages 1-8. McCarrison spent seven years as a physician among the isolated Hunza people, whose valley is now part of Pakistan. He saw no cases of cancer during that time, although, in those days, cancer was a well-recognized disease in Western countries. The Hunzas were so healthy that they rarely needed medical attention. McCarrison was able to spend his time doing research to find out why. He compared their diet to that of many other groups of people on the Indian subcontinent who weren't so healthy. Doing a large number of feeding experiments on mice, he was able to simulate in the mice the human illnesses characteristic of each group of people. He reached the conclusion that the secret of Hunza health was in their primitive diet.

But in recent times, the Hunza people have not fared well, for overpopulation in their valley forced them into eliminating cattle herds and cultivating all the land. Now a road into their valley brings outside commerce. They export some of their best foods, exchanging them for sugar, tea and other products. The Hunza now have many different health problems, including cancer. The long-lived people for which their valley became famous have all died off.

Certainly, every century has had its crusaders for healthy foods. But often, the message gets distorted. Thus yogurt is coming back as a health food, but the modern version is frequently so heavily sweetened that it should be considered a dessert. Also, some yogurts are pasteurized so that there are no viable lactobacillus in them. In memory of Sylvester Graham, we have graham crackers, but the modern versions of graham crackers have more white flour than graham flour. Graham flour is whole wheat flour plus extra bran.

A health-protective diet can also be an enjoyable diet. We don't really need most of the products of modern food technology. After you get used to whole foods, your taste buds will change. Thus the old-fashioned foods will seem tastier than the modern ones. You'll find that white bread tastes like cardboard, and you'll recognize when someone has laced your food with sugar or salt. Some of your old favorites are likely to taste too greasy. It will be a whole new world of food for you to explore with your "normalized" taste buds.

The best known guideline to foods, the Four Food Groups developed in 1955, is inadequate for optimum male health. To its credit, the guide does emphasize variety in its four main food groups: first is enriched or whole-grain bread, flour, cereals and potatoes; second is meat, poultry, fish, eggs and legumes; third is fruits (including citrus) and vegetables (including green leafy and yellow); and fourth is milk, cheese and ice cream. Some later versions deleted eggs from the list. Other versions have a fifth group of "foods" such as fats, sweets and alcohol. The guidelines were originally worked out to optimize intake of protein, five vitamins (A, C, B-1, B-2 and B-3), and two minerals (calcium and iron). But many essential nutrients have been discovered since, and new groupings of foods, based upon nutrient-density, are needed (see below). The Four Food Groups seem most suited to women of Northern European ancestry but are not even optimal for them. In this day of concerns for racial and ethnic equality, as well as for male health, it is time for drastic revision. The milk group should have less emphasis placed on it because so many have trouble with milk. Fruits and vegetables should not be put in the same class since fruits have a much lower nutrient density (though melons and tomatoes are on a par with many vegetables). Whole grain and "enriched" grain products are far different nutritionally, and thus should not be lumped together. (The word "enriched" is misleading, since two dozen nutrients were removed in processing and only four were put back in.) The Four Food Groups are too simple an answer with our present state of knowledge, and they fail as an educational tool.

Using the concept of nutrient-density, we can develop a far better ranking of foods. The foods with the highest nutrient-density are the most health-protective foods, in almost all cases. They have the most nutrients, or broadest spectrum of nutrients for the amount of calories.

The **first** rank on this scale would be certain vegetables and liver. These are almost complete in all nutrients. Some examples of vegetables with the highest nutrient-density are string beans, carrots, peas, cabbage, spinach, lettuce, or other fleshy or leafy vegetables. Yet, you couldn't live on those vegetables alone, for you would have to eat about 20 pounds per day to get enough calories. Strange as it may seem, liver is first rank, for it is lacking in only one nutrient, calcium. A few pounds of liver will give you a whole day's supply of calories. However, liver has too much vitamin A, so you shouldn't have a serving of it more than twice per week.

In **second** rank would be all the sources of high-grade animal protein: meat, fowl, fish, oysters, eggs and certain milk products. Men should only take fluid milk in their coffee or tea. Fermented milks, such as yogurt or kefir, are excellent. Strangely, when milk is converted to cheese, it loses much nutrient-density but becomes a protective food for men—an enigma for researchers to puzzle over. For vegetarians, legumes (dry beans, lentils and soybeans) combined with the right grains can provide reasonable protein.

Third rank would be whole grains, which are the best source of fiber and an important source of starch, along with vegetables like potatoes. Get variety in grains, selecting from wheat, rye, brown rice, corn, barley, oats, buckwheat, millet, etc. Whole grains keep well in storage, but the flours ground from the grains do not keep for long. (The oils in whole-grain flours go rancid quickly.   A good test is to put a sample of the flour on your tongue.   If you get a bitter taste, throw the whole lot away.)

Fourth rank would be fruits, which are a main source of vitamin C.   (Vitamin C tends to get cooked out of other foods.)   They are also a good source of bioflavonoids and certain useful fibers.   However, fruit fibers don't give much "bulking" action compared to grain fibers.

The **fifth** rank would be essential oils (polyunsaturates) from sources such as avocados, nuts, fish, peanut butter, mayonnaise, or extracted seed oils.   Only a small amount of oil is needed per day.   Vegetables may provide enough oil for some.   Butter can also provide some polyunsaturates.   All margarines contain too much modified oil to be used as a source of polyunsaturates.   Since extracted oils do not keep well, refrigerate, keeping away from air or warmth.

Most people get too much oil and not the right kind.   As mentioned previously, your diet should include a source of eicosapentaenoic acid (EPA), also called omega-3 oil.   If you eat quite a bit of fish that comes from cold waters, you won't need any more EPA as a supplement.   Taking EPA capsules is expensive and tedious, requiring up to 10 per day.   The easiest way to get your EPA is from food-grade linseed oil, available in health food stores.   Delicious salad dressings can be made from linseed oil, garlic and spices, and vinegar and/or lemon juice.   Make up a quantity and store it in your refrigerator. Lemon juice helps preserve the oil.

If you get a combination of these five ranks, you'll cover all nutrients in generous amounts.   The more of the four highest rank foods you get, the more protection you get against illness and disease.   Note that for men, milk must take a very low rank, because of its special problems, previously discussed. Your calcium will come from cheese, yogurt, dark green leafy vegetables, or certain ethnic foods like tofu or tortillas.   Also note that wilted, overcooked, canned or frozen vegetables have to go into a lower ranking than fresh ones.

There is another rank, which I'll call **bottom** rank. Mostly, they are the refined, partitioned, fractured or manu-factured foods.   You may eat modestly from this category, but only as a calculated risk. Nothing will happen to you right away, or for years, but over decades they may take a toll. The category includes most fats and oils, refined grains (white flour, white rice, degerminated corn meal), sugar, salt and alcohol. Within this lowest rank, we could identify some as not as bad as others—that is, some might have nutritionally redeeming features. Thus brown sugar is a bit better than white since brown sugar still has a full deck of minerals, though it has lost all vitamins, protein and fiber. On the other hand, honey has a broad spectrum of nutrients, but only in miniscule amounts and coming mostly from impurities such as pollen-grains. As to salt, it is better to use a salt that is a mixture of potassium chloride and sodium chloride, rather than ordinary salt.

We can make distinctions between different beers, too. In Olde England, beer was nutritious; and men survived mostly on dark bread, beer and some meat. They would hang any brewer who tried to speed up the brewing process by adding sugar to the vat, so they may have known of the unhealthy effects. Nowadays, it is good business practice to add sugar in brewing beer, since profits are increased. In the past, brewers have made other mistakes like fast-drying of the hops (which puts nitrites in beer), or adding cobalt to beer to give it more head (which killed a number of heavy beer drinkers through heart stoppage). A serious beer drinker should ask his brewer how the beer is made.

Descending further, nutritionally speaking, we have wine and hard liquor. Wine is replete with natural toxins left over from the fermentation, plus many dozen man-made additives allowed by law but not listed on any labels. Hard liquor has zero nutrient-density, but at least charcoal filtering may have taken out some toxic substances. The main toxin remaining is ethyl alcohol.

Besides food rank or nutrient density, there are other considerations. [Mertz '84] Variety in foods is important. Anyone who restricts himself to just a few foods, even the best of foods, or skips any of the top five ranks, is setting himself up for possible problems, either from deficiencies or from natural food toxins. As an example, suppose you want lots of cancer protection and go overboard on the recently touted cruciferous vegetables (brussel sprouts, cauliflower, broccoli and cabbage).   Unfortunately, these also have an anti-thyroid substance, so that you could end up with low thyroid function. At the other extreme, too much variety also carries a risk, since your taste buds may get overstimulated and lead you to overeat and put on weight.

Most people feel better and have more energy when they are getting some of the high-grade protein foods from animal sources: meat, fish, fowl, eggs, cheese or yogurt.   But those who get too many of the animal protein foods, with too few of the other protective foods, may be setting themselves up for trouble.   Vegetables provide important protective nutrients.

The time of day you eat food can make a difference.   If you tend to eat mainly one large meal per day in the evening, you may find a tendency to gain weight.   Those who skip breakfast, or just do a coffee and donut routine, are apt to find their energy flagging during the day.   If that is happening to you, try eating a high protein breakfast, and then concentrate more on the protective foods for the rest of the day.   You may be better able to experience all-day energy this way.

In general, the highly advertised foods are the worst. They have been the most tampered with nutritionally, losing nutrients and fiber, and gaining fat, sugar and salt.   They are also the most marked up in price.   So-called "fast foods" are not inherently bad, but the typical in fast foods (either in restaurants or in take-out foods) is close to the all-American diet—in other words, not all that healthy.   Fast foods tend to be weakest on vegetables and whole grains.   However, there have been notable improvements in some fast food restaurants offering salads and baked potatoes.   People in food businesses tend to offer what people want to eat.   Thus, if enough of you ask for whole grain bread or brown rice, sooner or later you'll find them offered.

It is not a good habit to eat unleavened bread, such as pita bread, whether made with whole or refined flour.   The advantage of yeast leavening is that it breaks down compounds called phytates, which can seriously bind up and prevent absorption of mineral nutrients.   The ideal period of yeast leavening is eight hours or more. Profit margins may lead many commercial bakers to shortcut this period.

You may have noticed in this book that I always refer to whole-grain bread, rather than whole-wheat bread. I believe there has been an overemphasis on wheat in our diets, to the detriment of people who tend to get allergies. Wheat is one of the most common allergies, outside of milk. If people got more variety in their grains, there would tend to be a bit less allergy to wheat. I recommend multigrain breads such as the seven- or nine-grain breads that can be found in health food stores and in some supermarkets. An allergy to wheat is likely to be due to either the gluten, or the germ. Sometimes bread made with sprouted wheat won't get an allergic reaction in people allergic to wheat flour.

Food allergy can complicate finding your own optimum nutrition. Such allergies can cause an extremely wide variety of symptoms. For those who might have allergies to a number of foods, blood tests may be the best way to help sort them out. Those on a budget could try a five day fast, at the end of which they'll probably feel great. They then reintroduce foods one at a time, testing their reactions. But if there are likely to be only one or two foods to which you are allergic, then it is fairly easy to experiment on yourself. What you have to do is note down your most common and favorite foods. One by one, you would avoid each food completely for at least five days (the time period necessary for that food to clear from your gut). Then eat that food alone while noting whether you develop any symptoms afterwards. One common allergic reaction is a sizable increase in your pulse rate about 30 minutes after eating a food. An increase of 15 or more beats per minute over your normal pulse rate suggests an allergy to that food.

We have to face up to some problems that can occur in the **transition** to a better diet. Allergy is of course one of these problems. Another is the gas or diarrhea that people experience when they increase their fiber intake suddenly. It takes your body some time to adjust to the increased fiber, but you and your gut will be far better off in the long run getting generous amounts of fiber, such as you would get from whole grains. Another of the problems in adjustment is that the extra fiber may cause you to lose minerals, especially zinc, during the interim period. Thus, multi-mineral supplementation may be needed (at least during the transition period). If you develop white spots on your fingernails, you know that you need extra zinc.

One error that some converts to whole foods make is to go to a health food store and start loading up heavily on food supplements like wheat germ, lecithin, brewer's yeast, nuts and seeds. These foods are good, but an excess of them gives you an excess of phosphorus, to the detriment of your body's calcium and magnesium status. Others start loading up on milk-based protein supplements, which is certainly unwise, especially for men. Loading up on bran, as separate from a properly leavened whole grain bread, also has the risk of carrying essential minerals out of the body.

Periodically, diet controversies erupt in the media, especially weight-loss diets. To invent a diet that is "new," one must go to extremes, such as extremely high protein, extremely low fat, all fruit, etc. The names of many diet proponents are best forgotten. Mostly, "crash" diets won't help you keep weight off for the long term, and may even contribute to later weight gain.

If you do try a high-protein diet, don't try getting **all** protein, such as in some of the liquid protein diets. These can kill. There must be vitamin and mineral supplementation with high-protein diets, as the leading proponent, Robert S. Atkins, M. D., amply points out. One of the more important nutrients that needs to be supplemented is magnesium. Also, the high-protein diet is not a long-term diet but a good temporary one if you are trying to drive fluid off your body quickly, or happen to be suffering from hypoglycemia.

The extremely low-fat Pritikin diet is one that many people find difficult to stick to. Such a low-fat diet tends to be unpalatable to many people. A low-fat diet tends to be a high-carbohydrate diet, and if the carbohydrates taken are whole and unrefined, it will also tend to be a high nutrient-density diet. The trouble with the Pritikin form of the diet is that it rejects some very nutritious foods such as liver, eggs, nuts, avocados, sardines, herring and shrimp——foods that we think of as appropriate in a healthy primitive diet. Cheese and butter are two other reasonable foods that are rejected. Pritikin also mistakenly rejected the use of vitamin and mineral supplements. His diet can produce abnormally low blood cholesterol levels, of unknown significance. To its credit, the diet appears to produce remarkably clean arteries, judging from the autopsy results on Nathan Pritikin. (See Chapter 11 for other information on low-fat diets.)

As to fruit diets, they have inadequate protein, so that the dieter ends up breaking down his own body proteins, including his muscles, in a form of self-cannibalism. My recommendation on diets is: don't wait for that magic new diet that will come out next week—just stick to the high nutrient-density foods, cut down on your total calories, get more exercise and take vitamin/mineral supplements.

* * *

You have to experiment to find what works best for you. Once you discover the best foods for yourself, you have won at least half the battle. Next let us go into greater depth on the problems of individual differences in nutrient needs, and the best ways of finding a practitioner to help.

CHAPTER 17

Individualized Nutritional Therapy

Throughout this book, I've commented on individual differences. You need only look at our faces to see that such exist. But then you'll also see resemblances within families. These same sorts of variations are found in our nutritional needs. Behind these themes with variations are our genes— which determine both physical appearance and nutritional needs. Each gene produces an enzyme. Thus, since families tend to share some identical genes, the amounts of each enzyme produced within family members will tend to be similar. The enzymes, both produced inside our bodies by the genes and supplied from without by food (i. e., vitamins), give us in turn a "network" of biochemical reactions. This network could be thought of as a multi-dimensional spider web, with each strand representing a chemical pathway.

Both the foods and the supplements we take provide enzymes from the outside. By adjusting diet or supplements, we can modify the balance of enzymes. This balance will help determine the "strands" of the web that will be emphasized. Of course, many enzymes will not get through various vital barriers inside your body. Your gut is one barrier protecting you from many "foreign" proteins; it will digest many of the enzymes. Sometimes, megadoses of a nutrient/enzyme will help a portion of the dose to get through.

If we have some genetic weaknesses or have had a less than optimal nutritional history, we can compensate somewhat by the level and the balance of nutrients that we put into our bodies. (The lifelong nutritional environment can also alter the potentialities of the genes.) But rather than attempt to use random experiment to determine the nutrients we need in extra amounts, we can use the results of tests, and also make some educated guesses. The hopelessness of doing random experiments with nutritional supplements can be appreciated if you consider that you might have to experiment with fifty different nutrients and various combinations of nutrients as well. It might take a lifetime of experiment to solve just one nutritional problem. Thus the optimum strategy with supplements is first to get a balance of all nutrients, note the results, then add on extra amounts of the nutrients that frequently help in the particular problems that you have.

The nutritional therapist will attempt to determine your biochemical pattern by various means. An analysis of your past diet is one piece of data. Another way to get insight is to look at your symptoms and past health problems, plus health problems of your parents and grandparents. Then there are measurements that can be made from blood, urine or hair samples. Blood and urine tests can be done for both vitamins and minerals. A sample of your head hair can be analyzed for minerals. [Passwater '83] In Appendix II, I've gone into some of the more important aspects of interpreting a hair mineral analysis. With our present state of knowledge, the interpretation of all the data is not usually clear-cut. To be safe, the nutritional therapist won't rely on a single piece of data but will look for a number of pieces all pointing in the same direction. It is all very much like detective work.

Roughly 1% of M. D.s are in nutritional practice. Many more are needed. There is very little to encourage physicians to go into the field, other than the desire to help their patients in the best possible way. It is difficult to get training in the field. Those who go into it may be ostracized and persecuted by their colleagues. Thus, when a nutritional M. D. effects a cure, his colleagues practicing conventional medicine are apt to call it a "spontaneous remission." More seriously, M. D.s are apt to have their license to practice questioned if they frequently use either vitamin B-12 injections or hair mineral analysis. It is also difficult for patients to collect on their medical insurance, for coverage may be denied either because it is "preventive" treatment or because it is not considered as being "conventional medical practice." The nutritional therapist can't run his patients through at the rate of 4 to 6 per hour, as in conventional practice, simply because there is just too much data for the nutritional therapist to gather and digest before reaching conclusions. Nutritional practice isn't likely to be a big money-maker for the physician.

Based upon objective scientific criteria, the practice of nutritional medicine is at least as well proven as conventional medicine. Strangely, the critics of nutritional medicine seem to demand that 100% of nutritional practice be supported by double-blind studies. That's a noble goal, but the critics forget that only 15% of conventional medicine is "proven," according to a 1978 report of the government's Office of Technology Assessment. That is about the same percentage as for nutritional therapy. Much of nutritional therapy does not lend itself well to double-blind studies because of the serious difficulties in selecting matched controls. It would be impossible to match people on all aspects of their nutritional state, which would include perhaps fifty different factors. Since genetic factors are usually important, one might also be limited to working with identical twins. Many excellent modern nutritional studies are based upon alternately giving and taking away the experimental nutrient on the same individual. Other nutritional therapy is based upon extrapolations from animal experiments.

If you wish to locate an M. D. of the nutritional specialty, you could check the yellow pages of your phone book where physicians are listed as to type of practice. There may be a listing of "Nutritional Medicine" or "Orthomolecular Psychiatry," or you may have to look under individual names to determine specialty. Word of mouth can help in locating a nutritional practitioner. Unfortunately, they are scarce in some parts of the country. Sometimes your county medical society can help, but you may be told that there aren't any nutritional therapists (if they aren't sympathetic to nutritional practice). Some books on nutritional therapy give a list of the many organizations that will help you in locating the right practitioner. (See bibliography in Appendix II.)

If you wish to have your nutritional status evaluated you can go to either an M. D. nutritional therapist or to a nutrition consultant. If you have possible serious health problems, you must see an M. D. first, for it is not legal for a nutrition consultant to diagnose disease. The quality of practice is certainly not standardized and, perhaps, it is just as well at the current state of knowledge of nutritional therapy. An M. D. may have just gone into the nutritional field and not be all that experienced. Ask about his experience in the field. If new to the field, he should be willing to research your case, and have the time to do it. This assumes that he has easy access to a medical library with the most important journals and books in nutritional medicine.

With regard to nutrition consultants, you must look into their background even more thoroughly. The fact that some-one has a diploma with the title "Nutrition Consultant" actually means nothing. You have to find out his relevant background in science and medicine. In a nutrition consul-tant, you most want to see a background in chemistry or biochemistry, and preferably some formal training in nutrition. Because the field is advancing so rapidly, someone who has an excellent scientific background, and who is willing to research your particular problems, could be better than a run-of-the-mill nutrition graduate.

There are many practitioners (including M. D.s, chiro-practors, homeopathists, nutrition consultants, etc.) out there claiming "alternative" or "holistic" medicine. These are two of the current buzzwords in therapy. Some of them may recommend rather unusual approaches to diagnosis and ther-apy. There are quite a few dubious therapies around. If a practitioner talks about the toxins in your body and suggests colonic irrigation, a fancy phrase for an enema, my advice is to hold your cheeks together and flee! Also, if the healer's background is in something like astrology, you might thank him politely for his time, excuse yourself and leave. If the practitioner seems to want to give you a lecture on health, rather than getting down to your specific health problems, you might want to find another. Don't be afraid to ask specific questions about a practitioner's background in, and specific approaches to, nutritional therapy.   Your health, your money, and your time are at stake.

In many ways, the individual must ultimately take charge of his own health, becoming expert on the needs of his own body.   To assist people in doing it right, there is Appendix II—Assessing Your Nutritional State.   It tells you about analyzing your diet, symptoms and signs, and the kinds of hard data you need.   It also tells how to interpret a hair mineral analysis.

*   *   *

The next chapter will cover the proper use of vitmain and mineral supplements, along with detailed information on the individual nutrients.

CHAPTER 18

Proper Use of Supplements

Whom are you going to believe? You've heard various experts say that all you have to do is to get variety in your food, that supplements aren't necessary, and that megavitamins are dangerous. Opinions may range upwards from the slightly negative "supplements can't hurt," to the slightly positive "supplements are good insurance," to the more enthusiastic "they'll do wonders for your health," and to the extreme view that huge doses are just right. Some say that synthetic vitamins are as good as natural ones, and others say you must take natural ones to get the benefits. And on and on it goes. The answer is, each of the experts has a piece of the truth but doesn't have the whole story. The problems we are running up against here are those of individual differences in needs, and of the impossibility of generalizing about all the nutrients.

Most of us hate to take pills. Thus we won't use supplements unless we see a good reason. Usually we have to be hurting first. But it is wise to remember that the physical symptoms of a health problem arrive in a late stage of a nutritional deficiency. The earlier stages include depletion of body stores, then biochemical abnormalities, followed by mental symptoms. [Brin '80] An excellent argument for supplements is that they may allow you to get away with a bad habit or two with less risk. Sometimes there are fairly immediate results upon trying them, but many of the benefits may be slow to appear. Thus it may be difficult to prove their value.

The net weight of all the amassed evidence indicates that supplements have benefits for most, if not all, people. Whatever, we are best off to use a **game theory** strategy here: There is a very small risk to taking supplements, and likely sizable benefits for long-term health.

Note that supplements are **not** a substitute for good food. But they may compensate partially for an inadequate diet. However, there are some people who, for genetic or other reasons, may need a quantity of one nutrient or another in amounts that they could never get from food. Finding out if you have any of these **nutrient dependencies** is an important step in reaching optimum health.

Here I hope to tell you the various ways to obtain and take supplements, leaving you to decide what will be easiest. There are all sorts of questions I hope to answer on dosages, when and how and which ones to take, whether to take multi-vitamin/mineral or individual nutrient tablets, whether to get synthetic or natural vitamins, and how to get high quality supplements at low prices. I also wish to warn you of interactions between supplements, and of dosages that might have side effects.

Should you obtain your supplements from a drug store, a health food store, or by mail order? Here is what I've found. Drug store supplements are frequently obsolete formulations, not up with the latest nutritional knowledge. Many supplements from health food stores are good formulations, but the prices are usually outrageously high. There is also a lot of pseudoscientific hype used in selling expensive supplements. I lean toward using a mail-order company, having found one that has both low prices and many good formulations. One good thing about a large mail-order house is that they tend to have a rapid turnover of their stocks, so that you can get the freshest possible supplements. (The potency of B-complex vitamins may be half-gone after a year or so on a store shelf.) You'll find mail-order houses advertising special prices in magazines such as "Prevention." The trouble with mail order is that you have to plan a week or two ahead of time.

If you appear to have no health problems, you may wish to take a multi-vitamin/mineral supplement for insurance only.

Then your body will select out what it needs from the supplement. If you are having health problems, or have a tendency to develop allergies, you'll want to be taking individual nutrient supplement tablets. It is more of a nuisance to take a load of separate pills, but then it is far easier to experiment with the supplements, to find out which help you the most, and to eliminate any that have adverse effects on you.

One problem in taking a large quantity of pills is that you feel bloated with water by the time you finish taking them. But there is a good trick to swallowing a whole load of pills, all at once, without even feeling them going down. You put them all on your tongue, work them to the back of your tongue, then take in a slug of water, tilt your head back, and as you swallow, bring your head back to level. Caution: practice this trick with one pill first, then work up in number as you gain confidence in the method. The trick will not work with lightweight pills that tend to float.

I see no reason to pay a far higher price for "natural" supplements than for synthetic ones. Besides, it is impossible to get sizable doses of many nutrients from natural sources. The biggest price rip-off is so-called "natural vitamin C," for it is 1% natural, 99% synthetic, and usually high priced. It is better and much cheaper to get synthetic vitamin C that has some bioflavonoids added. The bioflavonoids increase the effectiveness of vitamin C, and are always found with vitamin C in the natural state. Vitamins A, D and E are better in a natural form, unless the capsules have been around a long time and have become rancid. The word "natural," as applied to either foods, food supplements or vitamins is a highly misused or misleading word.

In recent years, much important nutrition research has had to do with the **interactions** of different nutrients. Because these interactions are so extensive, it is wise to get a balance of nutrients when you supplement. On top of that balance, you will then take extra amounts of those nutrients for which you appear to have an extra need. You make an educated guess as to which ones you have an extra need for, based upon what you've read in this and other books. Then you do a single experiment at a time—by taking one nutrient, or a group of nutrients that work together, in extra amounts, over and above a balance of nutrients. (See Appendix II.)

Now let us cover in greater detail the individual nutrients, including some of their interactions.

THE VITAMINS

Vitamin A: While cruising the South Pacific on a sailing yacht, I became somewhat of a miracle worker on a coral atoll, as I cured boils that had been festering for weeks. I also cured one child's troublesome earaches. My magic was vitamin A in a single dose of 25,000 i. u.   (I first took vitamin A along on my voyages to help prevent salt-water boils.) On a coral atoll, it is difficult to grow vegetables, and thus many people were deficient in vitamin A. While they ate considerable fresh tuna fish, they always threw away the guts, not knowing that a small piece of the liver would have been a potent source of vitamin A.

While vitamin A is best known for preventing night blindness, the above illustrates how important it is in combating infection. It is important to the health of all tissues, but especially of the skin and various mucous linings of the body. It is also helpful as cancer protection.

From the vitamin skeptics, you'll hear lots of warnings about overdosage. It is a bit tricky to tell whether there is a deficiency or an excess, for symptoms like hair loss or dry rough skin occur with either. You can get a severe headache from an overdose, or a sinus headache when you need more. Dosage of 200,000 i. u. daily for two months could produce vitamin A toxicity, but that dose for a few days could be therapeutic. The best way of protecting yourself from an overdose of A is to get good doses of vitamins E and C. You have to experiment to find your own optimum vitamin A dose, but it will probably range from 10,000 to 50,000 i. u. daily.

The two forms of vitamin A are retinol from animal sources and beta-carotene from plant sources. While the body is supposed to convert beta-carotene to retinol, it doesn't seem to do it efficiently in everyone. Too much beta-carotene will just turn your skin yellow, but too much retinol will give the toxicity signs. I lean toward taking the retinol form (from fish liver oil) because that happens to be what works for me.

B-complex Vitamins: You'll find B-complex tablets in dosages from RDA amounts (a few milligrams each of B-1, 2, 6, with a few micrograms of B-12) up to 150 milligrams of each. The better quality tablets will have as much B-6 as B-1, and tend to include up to 11 different B-complex factors.

Most characteristically, the B-complex factors help in nerve or nervous disorders, but can also help in a hundred other problems. You have to experiment to find the dosage levels that are best for you. If you are in poor shape from the all-American diet, you are apt to benefit from the higher doses. The most typical sign of an excess of B-vitamins is a headache, which could happen at ten times the RDA. Now we'll examine the individual B-complex factors.

Thiamine (B-1): Inadequate amounts of thiamine can lead to low energy, or to beri-beri. Not many cases of beri-beri are seen these days because refined grains are usually fortified with thiamine. Alcohol, drugs, stress and many other factors can deplete you of thiamine. If you have a magnesium deficiency, it may manifest itself as a seemingly high need for thiamine.

Riboflavin (B-2): Most of the problems found with a riboflavin deficiency are not especially unique to a riboflavin deficiency. But if you get cracks and sores in the corners of the mouth, a red sore tongue, or dry burning eyes, you might try riboflavin supplementation first. The fortification of refined grains with B-2 helps keep deficiency from being common, but there are some people with unusually high needs for riboflavin. Alcohol, drugs, stress and other factors can deplete you of riboflavin. When you take sizable doses of riboflavin, you are apt to notice that your urine becomes brightly colored.

Niacin, niacinamide (B-3):   Because most refined foods are fortified with niacin, the severe deficiencies of niacin which lead to pellagra are rarely seen.   The RDA for niacin is 18 milligrams.   Typical B-complex tablets have 100 mg. of the niacinamide form of B-3.   The niacinamide form is generally used in supplements, since 100 mg. of the niacin form can cause a skin flush reaction, which could be alarming to someone who doesn't expect it.   Megadoses of about 3,000 mg. niacin are used in some psychiatric disorders.   (You should be under the care of a physician to take such high dosages.)

Pantothenic acid (B-5):   The calcium pantothenate form is used in most supplements.   The National Academy of Sciences says that the "safe and adequate" dose of pantothenic acid is 4 to 7 mg. daily.   However, I've never heard of any problems with taking thousands of milligrams daily.   But start with 100 mg., and work up, finding the level which works best for you.   It's certainly a useful vitamin against stress, allergy and aging.   It can help some individuals recover lost ambition.   [Watson '72]   Refined foods cheat you of pantothenic acid.

Pyridoxine (B-6):   The RDA for vitamin B-6 is 2.2 mg.   But don't limit yourself to that amount unless you want minimum health.   It's my guess that about 10% of the population have a vitamin **B-6 dependency,** needing amounts that they could never get from food in order to maintain optimum health.   The extra need might range from 5 to 500 milligrams.   Be cautious with doses above 200 mg., for there can be serious side effects.   [Miller '82]   If you have white spots on your fingernails, it indicates a zinc deficiency, but extra B-6 may fix it up by promoting zinc absorption.   [Pfeiffer '78]

Vitamin B-6 can sometimes fix up a failing memory.   Your ability to recall your dreams when you wake up gives a good measure of your short-term memory.   Thus if you don't remember your dreams, or don't believe that you dream, try taking some vitamin B-6.   In fact, the amount you need is that which gives you reasonable dream recall.   If you take too much B-6, you'll be waking up too much from your dreams.

Vitamin B-6 can also help prevent atherosclerosis.   It

may do this partly by helping to break down homocysteine—a bad actor in your body—or by fostering magnesium uptake into your body's cells. An adequate dosage for this purpose is perhaps 25 to 50 mg. per day.

Almost always, you should supplement magnesium along with vitamin B-6. If you don't, you may find yourself getting irritable and having insomnia. The phenomena occurs because vitamin B-6 promotes uptake of magnesium by your body's cells (beneficially), but if you are somewhat short of magnesium overall, that will leave your blood magnesium low, and tend to overstimulate your brain.

There is an important interaction between vitamin B-6 and eicosapentaenoic acid (omega-3 oil), an oil that is rich in cold-water fish and in wheat germ and in linseed. If you have a vitamin B-6 dependency, you may find that it disappears after you get a teaspoon of linseed oil per day for a month. In fact, your body may no longer tolerate sizable B-6 supplements. [Rudin '82] Omega-3 oil may not take care of all the functions of B-6 in your body/mind, thus you may still need some extra B-6 supplementation.

Cobalamin (B-12): Since vitamin B-12 is found almost exclusively in animal products, strict vegetarians may have trouble getting enough B-12. Before pesticides were used, vegetarians had an easier time getting B-12, for there used to be enough insect parts in vegetables to supply enough B-12 to maintain health. This points up how small an amount of B-12 we actually need. The RDA is 3 micrograms (0.003 milligrams). Unfortunately, some people have a vitamin B-12 dependency which may come on insidiously with aging. The body's inability to utilize B-12 can lead to inadequate stomach acid being produced, pernicious anemia, or mental problems. In such cases, even large oral doses can not be adequately absorbed, so that vitamin B-12 injections are needed.

Biotin: Between dietary sources (liver and other high protein foods) and production by microorganisms in your gut, most people get adequate biotin (100 to 200 micrograms). But a few people have unusually high needs. Biotin deficiency can cause many different health problems.   Taking antibiotics can cause a biotin deficiency, but the gut flora can be restored by taking some yogurt.   If you are in the habit of eating raw egg whites, you are likely headed for trouble, for a protein in raw eggs will bind up biotin.   Cooked eggs are no problem.   The higher quality B-complex tablets contain some biotin.

Folic acid: High-powered B-complex tablets are relatively short on folic acid, for no tablet is allowed to contain more than 0.4 mg.(400 micrograms).   Thus extra folic acid tablets may be appropriate in order to achieve a better balance of the B-complex factors.   There are 0.8 mg. tablets available over the counter, labelled as being for pregnant or lactating women. (Don't let that bother you.)   In Canada, you can obtain 25 mg. tablets of folic acid over the counter.   The restriction on folic acid in vitamin supplements in the U. S. A. is intended to help doctors recognize cases of pernicious anemia.   If you have signs such as anemia, poor appetite, considerable weight loss, vague abdominal pains, burning tongue, or even temporary loss of sensations in the extremities, you should get checked out by a physician for the possibility of pernicious anemia, **before** you start taking folic acid supplements.

Choline: Choline is not fully accepted as an essential nutrient because there are chemical pathways for forming choline in the body by using other nutrients like methionine, folic acid and vitamin B-12.   But some people can't produce enough choline, so that dietary sources are advisable.   The best dietary sources are egg yolk or liver.   The better quality B-complex tablets will contain some choline, typically 250 mg. of choline bitartrate.   Choline is needed all over the body, but nowhere more than in your nerve fibers, where it helps form the sheaths covering the fibers.   It is also transformed into an important neurotransmitter substance, acetylcholine, which aids transfer of nerve impulses both to other nerve cells and to muscles.   Choline can help rescue some people from early senility or failing memory.

Inositol: The richest source of both choline and inositol is lecithin, which is helpful to some people with elevated blood cholesterol or triglycerides, or with heart disease.   If you take lecithin, be aware that it is loaded with phosphorus, and will thus increase your need for calcium and magnesium supplementation.   B-complex tablets with choline will usually include an equal amount of inositol.   Separate inositol tablets may be useful to some people who need tranquillizing or have insomnia.   Other nutrients could be helpful for these problems, too, such as magnesium, chromium, or tryptophan.

Para-aminobenzoic acid: Call this one **PABA** for short. Your body can convert PABA to folic acid if your diet is deficient in folic acid, and thus spare you from anemia.   While PABA may not be vitally essential, it may be essential for optimum health in some people.   It is included in the better B-complex tablets in 30 to 50 mg. amounts.   PABA is often used externally, especially in sun-screen lotions.

Vitamin C: The RDA amount of vitamin C, 60 mg., would appear to be intended to achieve minimum health.   Under stress, you need far more than 60 mg. of vitamin C.   Many men will find their optimum dose around 2,000 mg.   An excess of vitamin C will give you temporary diarrhea, but that usually requires a dose of about 5,000 mg.   While some experiments haven't shown the efficacy of sizable doses of vitamin C in preventing the common cold, experiments on men under heavy stress (such as soldiers out on bivouac) have shown highly significant results.

There are definite beneficial effects of 1,000 mg. or more of vitamin C on your blood lipids and clotting tendencies. [Bordia '80].

I must warn you that, after you have been on long-term vitamin C supplementation, you should not stop taking it, for you may get deficiency symptoms.   If you are planning to reduce vitamin C supplementation, taper off in your dosage over a period of a few months.

Vitamin C interacts with other nutrients.   It promotes the absorption of iron, and interferes with copper.   Because the all-American diet is short on copper, it would not be wise to take only vitamin C with such a diet.

Vitamin C has many different functions in maintaining human health. It is only man, the apes, monkeys and guinea pigs that are unable to produce vitamin C. All the other animals produce a quantity of vitamin C that is proportional to the amount of stress the animal is under. Mankind lacks a gene that produces an enzyme involved in the final step of vitamin C synthesis. Under stress, our bodies produce all the precursors to vitamin C but can't manage the final step.

Some experts warn you about the possibility of kidney stones if you take sizable doses of vitamin C. However, kidney stones are only a possibility in about 1% of people and could easily be prevented by supplements of magnesium and vitamin B-6.

Vitamin D: The RDA for adults is 200 i. u. If you are getting plenty of sunshine, there is no reason at all to get a vitamin D supplement. The sunshine in northern latitudes is adequate for whites, but not for blacks. Blacks living in northern latitudes should make sure that they get some vitamin D. There can be hazards in getting more than five times the RDA, unless you happen to be one of the rare individuals who need megadoses. Some people are allergic to the synthetic form of vitamin D which is called vitamin D-2, calciferol or irradiated ergosterol. The natural vitamin D is called vitamin D-3 or cholecalciferol, and generally comes from fish liver oil.

Recently, "experts" have been warning us to stay out of the sun or else use sun-blocking lotions because of the hazards of skin cancer or rapid skin aging. However, if you are practicing optimum nutrition, you needn't be quite so paranoid about sunshine.

Vitamin E: Typical American diets have been found to contain from 8 to 24 i. u. of **d-alpha tocopherol,** which is the most biologically active form of vitamin E. There are also other forms of vitamin E in food: beta, gamma and delta tocopherol. The delta form is the least biologically active, but has the best anti-oxidant properties. Anti-oxidants are important for your body, for they keep oils from turning rancid and protect your body's cells from free radicals. The best anti-oxidant nutrients are vitamins C and E and selenium. As a supplement, the best form of vitamin E is either the d-alpha form or the mixed form, containing alpha, beta, gamma, delta and some rarer types. To stabilize the vitamin E molecules, there is an acetate or a succinate group tacked onto the tocopherol. Although this isn't very natural, it is still called "natural" vitamin E and is an improvement over the truly natural. Any time that you see **dl-**, instead of just **d-**, in front of the **alpha,** you can be sure that it is synthetic vitamin E. I don't recommend large doses of synthetic vitamin E, for it will have extraction solvents remaining in it. If there is a preservative in your natural vitamin E, it may not be all that bad, for it will help keep capsules of vitamin E from getting rancid. And the fresher it is, the better.

Some foods lose most of their vitamin E during processing. Refined grains have lost almost all of their vitamin E, and frozen foods most of it. There are wide variations in cereals—corn flakes have lost all of their vitamin E, but puffed wheat and rolled oats keep most of theirs. But then, if the oats are cut or flaked, they lose it all. Overcooking or long storage will add to the losses. Oxygen is an enemy of vitamin E, either in food or in the body.

In the early space flights, the men ate freeze-dried foods and were breathing almost pure oxygen. During a flight, they lost about 25% of their red blood cells, becoming anemic, weakened and easily fatigued. On later flights, the food was supplemented with vitamin E, protecting the men. In a lack of sufficient vitamin E, particularly when breathing pure oxygen, all of the body's cell membranes are attacked by rancid oils and free radicals. Red blood cell membranes get weak and burst, and muscles start wasting.

Recent evidence shows that runners tend to become anemic, but cyclists don't. It appears that the pounding of the feet on the ground breaks red blood cells. There is no better way of protecting your red blood cells than by getting more whole foods and taking vitamin E supplements.

What sort of diet will give you the most vitamin E?

Richest in vitamin E are freshly-ground whole grains and sweet potatoes. Nuts, freshly shelled, are rich in E. Eggs are adequate, but meat has insufficient E (on a calorie basis). Milk is totally lacking. If you have much meat or milk, you actually need additional vitamin E to protect the sulfur amino acids, such as methionine. If your diet is rich in polyunsaturated oils, you need more vitamin E.

With the seeming impossibility of getting the ideal diet, and with air and water pollution increasing vitamin E needs, I recommend vitamin E supplementation. An insurance dose would be about 100 i. u. of the natural form. If you get no adverse side effects, a 400 i. u. capsule would be reasonable, especially in older people. (The dose of synthetic vitamin E needs to be larger to get the same effect.) As with vitamin C, you must not stop your vitamin E supplementation suddenly, or you are apt to get deficiency symptoms. The RDA, roughly 11 i. u., only insures minimum health. Besides, the RDA for adult humans was arrived at by extrapolation from the results of animal experiments, which are rather unreliable on vitamin E.

Vitamin E protects from all manner of problems of the circulatory system—short-lived red blood cells, excessive tendency of the blood to clot, varicose veins, hemorrhoids, intermittent claudication (pains in the legs while walking, due to muscles starved of oxygen because of narrowed arteries), atherosclerosis, angina pectoris (chest pains from oxygen-starved heart muscle), and coronary heart disease. Vitamin E reduces the oxygen requirements of oxygen-starved muscles. The required dosages may vary widely in different health problems. In rheumatic heart disease or congestive heart failure, the maximum safe dose might be 75 i. u. [Shute '77] In certain rare problems, the appropriate dose might range up to several thousand i. u. A physician should be involved in the treatment of most of the above-mentioned problems.

There can be side effects from vitamin E. A few percent of people get feelings of weakness or fatigue at doses above 100 i. u. Another small proportion of people may develop high blood pressure at 100 to 200 i. u. Some may get reduced thyroid or immune-system function above 400 i. u.

Vitamin E can also be useful externally, applied to burns,

sunburn, rashes, and leg ulcers.   It decreases pain, aids healing, and reduces scarring of the skin.

Essential Fatty Acids (EFA):   Some call this vitamin F. It includes polyunsaturated fatty acids.   These oils are mostly overused in the all-American diet, having been promoted as reducing blood cholesterol levels.   In Chapter 10 you learned that there are many other ways of reducing elevated blood cholesterol levels.   If you get too much of these oils, it can lead to reduced immune system function and possibly even cancer.   However, extra vitamin E should prevent excess oil from leading to cancer.   Excess oil can worsen gout.   As mentioned several times (for emphasis), the one oil that we need more of is omega-3 oil (EPA).

Vitamin K: Vitamin K is one of a number of factors that promote normal blood clotting.   A lack of it leads to inadequate clotting.   You'll get vitamin K in vegetables such as dark green leafies and broccoli.   You won't usually find vitamin K in supplements.   You can get shorted in vitamin K by not eating vegetables, through malabsorption of fats, liver problems, trying to eat a no-fat diet, or by taking antibiotics. Bacteria in your gut can produce vitamin K until antibiotics knock them off.   Symptoms of deficiency are easy bruising or nose bleeds, or worse.

Bioflavonoids: Although bioflavonoids are not accepted as essential nutrients, they are especially useful in enhancing the effects of vitamin C.   The pulp of citrus fruits is especially rich in bioflavonoids.   You can also take tablets.   A one gram tablet gives you as much as one orange.   Bioflavonoids help keep the walls of your small capillaries from breaking.   Those who bruise easily or get nosebleeds may need additional bioflavonoids, vitamin C, or vitamin K.

Pangamic Acid: This non-vitamin nutrient, sometimes called vitamin B-15, appears to help promote good tissue oxygenation and tends to fortify the immune system.   It is available as calcium pangamate, and the usual dosage runs 50 to 150 mg.   There appears to be a wide variation in the quality of the pangamic acid available.

THE MINERALS

Unfortunately, the public does not have much experience with mineral supplementation.   The only two minerals that have been emphasized much in the past are calcium and iron—two which answer to the needs of women but not of men. With mineral supplementation, the risks of side effects can be far greater than with vitamins.   To put it another way, the ranges of safe dosage are less than with vitamins.   Only rarely will you want to be taking a mineral supplement in much greater amounts than the RDA, for there is too great a chance of interfering with other minerals.   If you need to take two minerals that interfere with one another, you may circumvent the interference problem by taking supplements of the two interfering minerals at a different time of day or on different days.   If using supplements primarily for nutritional insurance (assuming there are no serious mineral deficiencies) a multi-mineral tablet is probably adequate.   Hopefully, your gut will select out and absorb the minerals that it needs most, although absorption will be inefficient.

Magnesium: Although I've covered magnesium already, there is much more that is important.   Deficiency causes health problems that develop insidiously.   Americans seem to be practicing "brinksmanship" with a diet so low in magnesium. Heavily strained are the body's abilities to retain magnesium. Because all sorts of stresses or bad habits cause loss of body magnesium stores, it's no surprise that many people get depleted of magnesium.

There are several possible interferences with other minerals.   There is a three way interference between calcium, phosphorus and magnesium.   Thus, if you have a diet of meat, milk, refined foods and phosphorus-loaded soft drinks, you'll be in trouble.   Doesn't that sound a bit like the all-American diet?   Another interference occurs between manganese and magnesium.   Thus in a diet short on magnesium, manganese would shove magnesium aside. But this interference doesn't occur often because American diets tend to be short on manganese, too.

Unfortunately, it is difficult to measure your body's magnesium levels. The most important measurement for men is a measure of heart muscle cell magnesium, since the heart muscle cells can get selectively depleted. However, it is not practical to take a biopsy while you are alive. Blood levels, either serum or red blood cell, may or may not show magnesium depletion. There is some hope in newer tests, one called a load test, and the other called a lymphocyte-magnesium test. [Flink '80, Cohen '83]

There is a long list of possible symptoms of magnesium deficiency. Unfortunately, the symptoms are not particularly specific. Signs or symptoms that can suggest magnesium deficiency are: insomnia, tension, being overly keyed up, jumpiness at the slightest noise, anxiety, muscular twitching or tetany, tremors, convulsions, excessive sweating or body odor, vertigo (dizziness), memory impairment, apathy, depression, confusion or disorientation, paranoia, involuntary hand movements, difficulty in swallowing, heart arrhythmia, angina, congestive heart failure, stupor or coma, nystagmus (involuntary rapid oscillating eye movements), hallucinations (usually visual), etc. If you have a number of these signs, there is a good chance that you are magnesium deficient, or have a depletion of body stores. In some cases, the first overt signs of magnesium depletion can be changes in the electrocardiogram, a heart attack, or sudden cardiac death. Some drugs may contribute to depleting you of magnesium, such as antibiotics, diuretics, and digitalis.

The opposite problem, magnesium excess, can be seen in cases of kidney failure. It can also be seen with excessive supplementation with magnesium. The most likely symptoms would be lethargy, unexcitability and a slow heart rate. [Graber '81, Mordes '77]

The proper amount of magnesium supplementation you should get each day depends drastically on the type of life you lead and the foods you eat. If you have been on the all-American diet, you should add 200 to 300 mg. per day. If you have been on the all-American diet and living life in the fast lane, with assorted bad habits, you should add something like 500 mg. per day.   If you eat whole foods and lead a fairly stress-free life, you may not need any extra magnesium. Along with magnesium supplementation, it would be wise to get 25 to 50 mg. per day vitamin B-6 to help the magnesium get into your cells.   The usual magnesium supplements are magnesium oxide or dolomite (which has calcium, too).   If you take chelated magnesium, you won't need quite as much supplemental magnesium.   The best absorbed magnesium supplement is probably magnesium aspartate.   If you have digestive problems, especially low stomach acids, you'll especially need the chelated forms.

Calcium: Many Americans tend to get a poor balance of minerals from their diet.   The excess salt that many consume tends to increase the loss of calcium through the urine.   To make up for this loss, rather than supplementing heavily with calcium, which would then work against your magnesium status (through the calcium-phosphorus-magnesium interference), it is best to cut back on salt.   The extra calcium would also work against your zinc and manganese status through another type of interference.

However, if you get too little calcium, you are setting yourself up for high blood pressure and a stroke, unless you cut down on your salt and get more magnesium in your diet (as would be found in a typical primitive diet).

Perhaps now you are beginning to see how complicated it gets when you have nutritional imbalances.   But don't start worrying too much about balance.   Your body can tolerate minor imbalances if you get enough of all the essential nutrients so that regulatory mechanisms can work efficiently.

The RDA for calcium is 800 mg. per day.   You should try to get that through the sources given in Chapter 9—cheese, yogurt, greens, tofu, beans, tortillas—preferably avoiding milk.   However, if you are allergic to cheese or yogurt, you can expect to need calcium supplementation.   Oyster shell, egg shell calcium or chelated calcium are probably the best supplements.   If you take in 800 mg. of calcium, then you ought to get about 500 mg. magnesium. However, if you get lots of yogurt and little salt, then a higher calcium to magnesium ratio should be safe (as it is with the Masai, an extreme case). There appear to be considerable individual differences in calcium needs, some needing more like 1200 mg. per day. However, the apparent extra need for calcium may disappear when the rest of the diet is improved.

Sodium and **Potassium**:   I'm covering these two together because of their mutual interference with one another.   If you get too much sodium, it will adversely affect your potassium status, and vice versa.   Refined foods that have salt added are good examples of what not to eat.   They've lost their potassium and magnesium, and gained sodium, making them a one-way ticket to imbalance.   If you are going to salt your food anyway, you might switch from using sodium chloride to using a salt that is a mixture of potassium chloride and sodium chloride.   It is readily available in your supermarket.

A shortage of potassium will generally lead to muscle weakness.   Sometimes the body can't hold on to potassium because of magnesium depletion.   Most of the potassium in your body is **inside** the cells.   Thus, if you are having a blood test done, it should be red blood cell potassium rather than the usual test of blood serum potassium.

In contrast, sodium is mostly **outside** your cells, in your blood serum or in your gut.   There are some people who appear to need a sizable sodium intake, just as there are others who can't tolerate much sodium without bloating up or getting high blood pressure.   Those who work in a hot environment are likely to need some extra sodium and other minerals.

Zinc and **Copper**:   There is a strong mutual interference between these two trace elements.   Since zinc supplementation has become popular, there have been numerous people who have driven their copper levels down.   Note that large doses of vitamin C can also drive copper levels down.   A diet of refined foods is seriously lacking in copper, but you could get enough copper if you have copper plumbing in your home.   A copper lack can contribute to numerous problems, including irregular heart beat, high blood cholesterol, ulcers and gout. [Klevay '82, '80]   Arthritis can result from either too little or too much copper, but there are other possible nutritional factors in arthritis.   Women are far more likely to have high copper levels than men, but in a man a high copper level is likely to lead to hyperactivity.   Zinc supplementation is the best way to bring a high copper level down.

The ideal ratio of zinc to copper in a supplement for someone in reasonable balance is about ten to one, but the ratio can vary between 7 and 15.   In other words, a reasonable supplement might be 20 mg. zinc and 2 mg. copper.   If you are depleted of both zinc and copper, you must take the zinc and copper supplements at different times of day for the best effect.   Also, note that folic acid supplements can interfere with zinc absorption.   Thus, if it is important that you get zinc supplementation, take zinc tablets a half-day separated from folic acid tablets.

People with white spots on their fingernails need zinc supplementation.   Thirty to fifty milligrams of zinc daily (possibly higher initially) plus 25-50 mg. of vitamin B-6 would be appropriate for most cases.   Others with zinc deficiency, or extra need for zinc, are a bit harder to identify, but tell-tale signs are a history of eczema (a skin condition), slow maturation in young men, or prostate problems in older men. Therapeutic doses of zinc of 150 mg. or so are sometimes used but are usually not necessary when vitamin B-6 is taken as well.   The side effects of excess zinc dosage are most likely to be lethargy, nausea or diarrhea.

Zinc is excellent for helping to drive out some of the toxic metals, such as lead and cadmium.

Iron: Maintaining your iron status at a reasonable level gives you more physical energy.   The usual blood tests for iron are not all that useful, except in outright anemia.   The best test of tissue (cellular) iron stores is serum ferritin.

Men don't tend to need much iron supplementation; the RDA of 10 mg. should be adequate for most.   Women aged 15 to 50 need about twice as much.   The supplement should be the **ferrous** form of iron, not the **ferric** form, which is useless.

There are a number of different minerals that, in excess, will interfere with your iron status: manganese, zinc, cobalt, phosphorus and potassium.   Vitamin C is very helpful in promoting iron absorption, as are copper and nickel.   Oddly, excess copper works against iron.   Heavy tea and coffee habits can work against iron absorption.

Manganese: Most Americans, as compared to people of the less developed nations, are low in manganese.   The reason appears to be our methods of fertilizing the soil, which cause our vegetables to be short in manganese.   (Vegetables grow well without manganese.)   The minerals that interfere with the manganese status, of either your vegetables or your body, are calcium, potassium and phosphorus.   [Davies '72]   Farmers among you will recognize the components of modern agricultural fertilizers.

There can be subtle health problems that develop when you are short on manganese.   Because manganese aids the utilization of B and C vitamins, someone short in manganese will find benefit in sizable doses of the B and C vitamins. Manganese levels can only be restored over a lengthy period (years).   Supplements aren't well retained by the body but are still worthwhile in the amount of 5 to 25 mg. per day. English-type tea is the richest dietary source of manganese.

Chromium: The typical American has low body stores of chromium.   Chromium is extremely important for proper blood sugar regulation.   Its lack is associated with atherosclerosis, hypoglycemia or diabetes.   Contributing to a body shortage of chromium are factors such as American soils being depleted, food refinement, and foods that tend to use up body chromium stores.   Eating sugar or taking sweet drinks tends to cause chromium loss through the urine.   The phosphorus in milk tends to bind up and make useless the chromium in food.

Among chromium supplements, GTF-chromium is by far the most useful one, for it is well absorbed and utilized.   A maintenance dose of GTF-chromium might have 50 mcg. elemental chromium, while a therapeutic dose would have 200 mcg. or more.   Many chromium supplement tablets contain inorganic chromium or chelated chromium. Unfortunately, this chromium is poorly absorbed by those who need it most.

Selenium: It looks like selenium helps protect you from both cancer and heart disease. The exact connections are the subject of much research at present. A safe and adequate dose of selenium is considered to be 50 to 200 micrograms. Selenium is toxic at levels of 500 to 1,000 micrograms daily. In some parts of the Midwest and the Rockies, the soil and water are rich in selenium and it would be unwise for the people to take any supplementation. The East Coast soil tends to be short on selenium, and so supplementation of perhaps 100 micrograms makes good sense.

Iodine: Iodine will be found in seafood, kelp, and in most multimineral supplement tablets. If you get too little iodine, it can lead to goiter. Goiter usually only occurs in inland areas where the iodine has been leached out of the soils, and among people who avoid seafood. However, some people have a problem with even modest supplements of iodine, which may cause them to break out with acne.

Nickel, vanadium, molybdenum, silicon, tin, fluorine and **arsenic**: These trace elements have been found to be essential, but only in tiny amounts. They are not usually found in supplement tablets—especially arsenic, since it is toxic at fairly low levels. You'll find sufficient of these minerals in whole foods but not in refined foods. Deficiency experiments performed on small animals can show some rather bizarre effects. But it is impossible to do the same experiments on an animal as large as man, because it takes many years to deplete a large animal, and it might even take a generation or two for the problems to show up.

* * *

Once more, I must emphasize that you are playing Russian roulette with your long-term health when you eat refined foods, for you'll be cheated of both vitamins and minerals.   The subtle physical and psychological ailments you develop will not seem to have much relation to your nutrient intakes, until after you get rid of the ailments by increasing nutrient intakes.   On refined foods, for example, your body may no longer be able to regulate its mineral levels properly. You may absorb toxic metals, and/or end up with mineral imbalances—different imbalances in different people.

CHAPTER 19

Beating the Odds

By now, it should be clear how you can beat the odds against you—using nutritional knowledge. Possibly you can keep some of your bad habits, and stop worrying or feeling guilty about them. Even though your supposed chances of getting heart disease are three times as high if you smoke or lead a stressful life, or about twice as high if you are a heavy drinker, you know that those figures apply to the fellow with average nutrition—the all-American diet. If you practice optimum nutrition and take the appropriate supplements, you should be able to reduce the risks considerably.

If an "expert" warns you about your habits, you can just smile. You're one step ahead of him. To protect his facade, he'll tell you: "But the case for optimum nutrition and taking supplements isn't proven yet." He really means it isn't "generally accepted" within the ideological framework of the medical system. Just tell him that you want to take a game theory approach to it, that the possible benefits are large and the risks small. Remind him that you can't wait 50 years for absolute proof—it would be too late for you then, and you want to have a long, healthy and happy life. If the expert persists, put him on the defensive with the fact that only 15% of conventional medical practice is proven, according to a 1978 Office of Technology Assessment report.

One of the ideologies of the medical system is that you can get all the vitamins and minerals you need from eating a variety of foods. Naturally, dieticians are trained to believe this ideology. Yet a recent poll of dieticians revealed that a majority of them take vitamin and/or mineral supplements. If dieticians don't even follow what they are taught (and teach), why should you believe what the medical system teaches? Of course, the medical system is not one voice, but many. Quite a few physicians already accept the need for supplementation, but don't know enough about proper use. The problem goes back to medical education, in which nutrition gets short-changed.

Mostly, I've concentrated in this book on what the individual can do for his own health. But some words need to be said about how badly messed up the medical system is. If you keep yourself in optimum health without recourse to health facilities, you may get the mistaken impression that you aren't paying for the system. Consider that an eighth of your federal, state and local taxes goes to health care. Additionally, if your employer provides health benefits, you are paying for that as well, although indirectly. But that is not the worst news, for the trend in future costs are really alarming. The medical system is gobbling up a greater and greater proportion of the economic "pie" as time goes on, and promises to become an incredible burden on all of us. Medical costs nearly double every five years. They are now almost 11% of the gross national product of this country.

Some say the medical cost increases are caused by people living longer. While that may be true for costs of the Social Security system, it should not be a factor in health costs. The problem is more likely to be in the cost of degenerative diseases, rampant in Western countries, but almost absent in the least developed countries. In the healthiest primitive societies, the aged tend to maintain good health up to near the end. Like the one horse shay, they tend to break down rapidly shortly before death. A forecast for the year 2000 by the Institute for Alternative Futures suggests that there will be a nine-year difference in male/female life expectancy in this country. Men will only be spared by a rethinking of their food habits and by nutritional supplements, along the lines suggested in this book. Women will also be helped, but male life expectancy will be boosted more.

Over a 15-year period, a poll showed that the proportion

of people generally trusting physicians went from 73% down to 30%. The greater number of people suing their doctors also shows this loss of confidence. Many doctors make the mistake of projecting too much authority and self-confidence. (It's part of the laying-on-of-hands, which helps get "placebo" cures.) However, it is clear that doctors only deserve a small part of the blame for the problems. They are caught in the middle, with medical malpractice insurance rates skyrocketing. Our legal system forces doctors to practice defensively, ordering extra tests and doing extra paperwork, to protect their rear flanks. Of course, some law suits result from physician malpractice, but at least as many stem from the relative ineffectiveness of much of conventional medicine. I believe that the practice of nutritional medicine will help get doctors out of a bind, bringing better and longer-lasting cures, requiring more contact with the patient (which inspires a more genuine trust), and allowing the doctor to level more with the patient.

It would be easy to blame the medical profession for slowness to change, the legal profession for venality, the food industry for opportunism, the people for buying and eating junk (and expecting too much of medicine), or the government for its bureaucratic tangles. More fairly, we might blame the so-called civilized society which we seem to have evolved. Or, more basically, we might admit that we need to improve the way in which individuals relate to one another. As indicated previously, nutrition can influence our mental well-being, and therefore our ability to relate to others amicably. However, many factors other than diet work against us. For instance, experiments have shown that noise makes people uncaring about their fellow man. Crowds and cities also make people uncaring. Still, we must reckon that the long-term dietary drift that has occurred contributes to a significant share of our interpersonal problems.

*   *   *

First let me summarize the shifts needed in our food habits:

1.   Milk should be processed more, into cheese or yogurt.
2.   Grains should be processed less, that is, should be

unrefined, and include the bran (fiber) as well. Because of the limited shelf life of whole grain flours, consider buying the grains and grinding them yourself on an inexpensive electric grain-grinder.

3. Eat more vegetables and salads, especially if you've been neglecting them.

4. Ease off on using most oils, but get some omega-3 oil (EPA) into your diet. This will involve eating some fish (especially cold-water fish) or the use of linseed oil, perhaps by making your own salad dressing with it.

5. Limit your intake of sweeteners to small amounts spaced out over time.

6. If you are going to continue using a salt shaker, at least use a salt that is a mixture of potassium chloride and sodium chloride. Generally avoid foods loaded with sodium chloride.

These modest shifts will bring you close enough to the primitive whole-food diet, and take you far enough away from flaming out.

Now let me summarize the general range of daily vitamin and mineral supplementation that you'll probably find optimal:

> Vitamin A, 10,000 to 50,000 i.u. (Dosage in the upper part of the range should be accompanied by vitamin E and C supplements. Women who are pregnant must avoid sizable vitamin A doses.)
>
> B-complex tablet, from RDA amounts up to a "B-50" tablet
>
> Extra folic acid, vitamin B-6, or pantothenic acid, as needed
>
> Vitamin C, 1,000 to 5,000 mg., preferably with some bioflavonoids
>
> Vitamin D, 200 i.u., but none if you get much sunshine
>
> Vitamin E, 100 to 400 i.u., in either the "d-alpha" or "mixed" tocopherol form

Magnesium, 100 to 500 mg. supplementation, depend-
    ing upon diet and lifestyle.   Men need more
    than women.
Calcium, total daily intake of 800 mg., from both
    food and supplements.   (Women may need
    additional calcium.)
Zinc, 10 to 30 mg.
Copper, 1 to 3 mg.
Iron, 10 mg. for men, and 18 mg. for women
Manganese, 5 to 15 mg.
Chromium, 50 to 200 micrograms, from GTF-
    chromium
Selenium, 0 to 150 micrograms, depending upon your
    diet and in what part of the country you live

(The above figures assume that you don't have special
health problems.   Of course, dosages must be tailored to the individual situation; and therapeutic
doses may be higher.   See other chapters for more
complete details.)

                        *   *   *

If you can practice a bit of nutritional self-discipline to
overcome the innate tastes (for sugar, salt and fat) that lead
us astray, and heed the lessons in this book about the problems
of milk and refined grains, then you'll be well on your way to
preventing health calamities in your life.   As added insurance,
at modest cost and effort, it is wise to get in the habit of
taking vitamin and mineral supplements.   You will also do well
to encourage others around you to improve their nutritional
habits.   Hopefully, it will bring about better health and lower
medical costs for all of us.

Here's to your optimum health!

Toward a Unified Hypothesis of Coronary Heart Disease

Medical researchers desperately need a newer, broader and more valid **conceptual framework** in which to fit the great mass of data on coronary heart disease (CHD).

Consider the lengthy list of theories of the origins of CHD, and risk factors for CHD, which could reasonably include:

1. excessive dietary fat and cholesterol
2. atherosclerosis
3. stress (type "A" behavior; emotional distress)
4. smoking
5. elevated blood cholesterol
6. coronary artery spasm
7. arrhythmia
8. homocysteine theory
9. altered prostaglandin metabolism
10. enhanced blood platelet aggregation
11. smooth muscle degeneration in the arteries
12. balance of sex hormones
13. low testosterone level in males
14. high level of LDL or low level of HDL
15. modified oils in diet
16. lack of certain oils in diet
17. allergy
18. virus
19. low thyroid function
20. genetic predisposition

21. environmental pollutants (Pb, CO, CS_2, etc.)
22. damage by free radicals
23. nutritional deficiencies
24. nutritional imbalances
25. high blood pressure
26. heavy drinking
27. obesity
28. lack of exercise
29. excessive exercise
30. lack of dietary fiber
31. excessive sugar
32. excessive calories
33. diabetes
34. age
35. high blood triglycerides
36. chlorine in drinking water
37. soft (or softened) drinking water
38. coffee
39. liquid protein diets
40. high dietary ratio animal/vegetable protein
41. pasteurizing of cows' milk
42. xanthine oxidase in homogenized milk
43. lack of negative air ions

If I've forgotten a few, I wish to apologize to the researchers involved! I'm inclined to accept all of the theories/risk factors as being valid contributors to CHD. I assume that the researchers are competent and have only the best of motives. Each case of CHD probably has at least several main causes and a number of minor contributing factors. Different cases will have a different mix of factors. If most cases of CHD in this country have a limited number of causes, and mostly the same causes, then there is a possibility for mass prevention through education or public health measures. If not, then individual treatment will be of primary importance. The evidence presented in this book suggests that there are some main causes in common, but that there are also individual factors. Thus a combination of mass and individual measures will be most successful.

The research on CHD has led to many heated controversies. [Nutrition Today '84, '80] These controversies stem from the inherent complexity of CHD. As a most important step in trying to resolve the controversies, it is necessary to examine the underlying metabolic mechanisms (as best as they are known) of each of the theories/risk factors. Even a cursory examination of the list shows a number of them to be interrelated. However, we don't know the detailed mechanisms of many of them, so that the process of forming a valid conceptual framework is made more difficult.

Having looked into some of the metabolic mechanisms, I'm convinced that the data can be integrated best using knowledge from the field of nutritional biochemistry, with some assist from molecular biology. No doubt there will be much resistance to this idea from medical researchers who have not had extensive experience in these areas.

If in this book I have been harsh in my criticisms of the fat-cholesterol hypothesis and the risk-factor approach to CHD, it is because I feel that they have been overpromoted, to the exclusion of other theories that are at least as valid. The fat-cholesterol hypothesis has to be considered a poor working hypothesis, since 35 years of major effort have not led us to any definitive experimental results that can lead to the elimination of CHD. The data coming out are interesting enough but seem only marginally relevant to the task of eliminating CHD. There have been many elaborate studies, conducted in a wide variety of countries, to test the risk-factor approach to CHD. Mostly the studies have to be considered as less than successful. [Enloe '84, Kolata '85, Oliver '83] Neither the fat-cholesterol hypothesis nor the risk-factor approach can have a central position in a new conceptual framework for looking at CHD. Still, they must be considered as contributing factors.

The results of two different animal experiments give us a strong clue that the conceptual framework must be centered upon nutritional factors other than fat and cholesterol: (1) In rabbits fed sizable quantities of fat and cholesterol, atherosclerosis develops, but not if the rabbits are also provided with magnesium. [Neal '62]; (2) In simulating human-like heart attacks in rats, the diets used by J. Sós and coworkers were fairly low fat, about 21% on a calorie basis. The feeding of saturated fat, rather than unsaturated, did not have a significant effect on rat heart deaths. Leaving cholesterol out of the cardiopathic diet reduced the death rate by 30%, but omitting the mineral imbalances (high Ca/Mg and high Na/K) reduced the death rate by 85%. [Sós '65] Thus mineral imbalances are likely to be of more importance than dietary fat and cholesterol. Because of the interactions between lipid and mineral metabolism, in which minerals are beginning to appear more important, the cholesterol-feeding experiments on humans must be repeated with minerals (and vitamins) taken into account. Until repeated, all the cholesterol-feeding data is suspect.

There is one telling argument against current approaches to CHD. Commenting on the recent results of the National Heart Lung and Blood Institute's (NHLBI) Lipid Research Clinic CHD Primary Prevention Trial (LRC-CPPT), in which a drug that lowers blood cholesterol levels was used, Michael F. Oliver, of the University of Edinburgh, said: "It should not be too surprising that CHD death rates are unaltered since a number of the mechanisms leading to death have nothing to do with raised cholesterol levels (e. g., ventricular fibrillation, acute thrombosis, coronary spasm)." [Oliver '84]

Similarly, we can say that all the risk factors so heavily emphasized (i. e., blood cholesterol levels, atherosclerosis, elevated blood pressure, low HDL, high LDL, smoking, drinking, type "A" behavior, lack of exercise, obesity, dietary fat, and dietary cholesterol) are only **indirectly** related to the events that occur just prior to a CHD death.

But all three of the above-mentioned precursors to a CHD death—ventricular fibrillation, acute thrombosis, or coronary artery spasm—can be produced by common nutritional imbalances. Consider that magnesium depletion can contribute to all three. [Flink '81, '78; Dyckner '80, Ghani '77, Iseri '75, Loeb '68 (as to ventricular fibrillation); Szelenyi '73, Vivier '79 (as to acute thrombosis); Turlapaty '80, Altura '79 (as to coronary artery spasm)] Magnesium is of such importance that three major works have been published on it.

[Cantin '80, Seelig '80, Wacker '80]   Reviews of magnesium are apt to have titles like, "The Forgotten Electrolyte" or "The Neglected Cation."   [Bigg '80, Flink '80, Geiderman '79, Graber '81, Seelig '74]

Because factors other than magnesium depletion can contribute, the new conceptual framework must not be limited to magnesium depletion.   As an example, consider that all of the following nutritional factors help reduce excessive platelet aggregation (which is probably a main contributor to acute thrombosis): vitamin C, vitamin E, vitamin B-6, magnesium, eicosapentaenoic acid (omega-3 oil), and substances in pineapple (bromelain), garlic and onions.   [Martin '83, Bordia '80] Additionally, the new conceptual framework must not be limited to nutritional deficiencies and/or nutritional imbalances, for environmental pollutants are also likely to play a part. As mentioned previously, I found toxic levels of lead in the hair of two out of eight cases of sudden cardiac death.   If we concentrate on the underlying metabolic mechanisms, it will help us avoid oversimplifying, and allow a way to integrate all of the various theories and risk factors of CHD.

Integrating the fat-cholesterol hypothesis into the new framework should not be difficult.   After all, there are about 20 different nutrients or food factors that will lower the blood cholesterol level (listed in Chapter 10).   In Western countries, excessive dietary fat and cholesterol may well be a contributor to CHD, but mainly because of some other dietary imbalances that disturb cholesterol metabolism.   In people who have not been "westernized," such as the Masai, it is clear that dietary fat and cholesterol are not a factor in CHD.

Integrating risk factors into the new framework can be managed if one considers that many of these factors either interfere with biochemical functions that are part of the body's normal repair and protective mechanisms, or disturb regulatory mechanisms.   (More than biochemistry is needed in explaining arrhythmias, for electrical phenomena must be taken into account.)   Moreover, some of the risk factors are known to have anti-nutrient effects, so that the connection to nutritional deficiencies or imbalances is readily made.

Another useful way of looking at the problem of CHD is

that there need to be enough protective nutritional factors in the diet to prevent damage by the risk factors. Diets in Western countries have lost a large portion of these protective nutrients through refinement of foods.

There is considerable support, in both recent worldwide data and the 1920-1985 U. S. A. data, for a conceptual framework based upon nutritional factors. Review Figure 2 on page 41, and also recall that in the U. S. A. the dietary ratios of both calcium to magnesium and of sodium to potassium peaked in the 1960's when CHD deaths peaked. [Friend '79, '67; Marston '81] A framework of this sort could most appropriately be called an electrolyte-derangement hypothesis. [Raab '69] There is also good support for nutritional factors from both animal experiments and human clinical data, especially for magnesium. [Seelig '80, Browne '63, Davis '78, Malkiel-Shapiro '60]

Because smoking peaked about the same time as the dietary ratios of calcium to magnesium and of sodium to potassium, it could be argued that smoking must also be considered as an important factor. However, we have to note the hard-to-explain fact that smoking associates much more strongly to myocardial infarctions than to brain infarctions. [Kannel '85] While that fact is not understandable in terms of a "smoking" hypothesis, it fits in beautifully with an "electrolyte derangement" hypothesis. It fits because calcium is protective against strokes, but appears to promote myocardial infarctions (through either a high dietary calcium to magnesium ratio, or through adverse factors in the skim milk fraction, as discussed in Chapters 7 through 9). Thus smoking, the "prima donna" of the conventional risk factors, may have to take a back seat to electrolyte derangement as a risk factor.

As to the decline of CHD deaths in the U. S. A. during the past two decades, there is a good chance that it has something to do with shifts away from milk, toward cheese and yogurt, toward less refinement of grains, towards less use of salt, and toward greater use of vitamin and mineral supplements. Medical interventions may also have contributed in the past decade or so, with coronary care units, increasing knowledge of cardiopulmonary resuscitation, control of high blood pressure, and other advanced techniques.

It is encouraging that the nutritional factors mentioned as likely to be major contributors to CHD lend themselves well to mass educational efforts. Additionally, only minor change in our basic food supply is required to eliminate much of CHD. The needed changes are mainly in the processing of food. Specifically, grains must be processed less, and milk processed more. Most other schemes to reduce CHD would require drastic upheavals in U. S. agriculture.

All of the medical literature I have reviewed appears to support the scheme of Figure 2, except for one single paper. But that paper is balanced off by a paper with an opposite finding. In cholesterol-fed rabbits, Kiyosawa found that skim milk produced no atherosclerosis, but that whole-milk yogurt did produce some atherosclerosis. [Kiyosawa '84] It isn't clear to me why he compared whole-milk yogurt to skim milk, rather than comparing skim-milk yogurt to skim milk. That would seem to be loading the dice against yogurt, since the rabbits in the yogurt group would be getting more fat. Earlier, Thakur performed similar experiments and found yogurt to be more protective than milk against both atherosclerosis and hypercholesteremia, but did not mention whether or not the milk and yogurt were skim or whole. [Thakur '81]

In light of Terpstra's careful review of the subject of cholesterol and the protein feeding of animals, in which there appears considerable variability in results, depending upon animal species and type of protein fed, I would conclude that **none** of the rabbit data could be safely extrapolated to man. [Terpstra '83] I firmly believe that it is far better to work with an omnivorous species like the rat, as did Sós, stimulating human-like myocardial infarctions and sudden cardiac death. [Sós '65] Otherwise, one is making too many extrapolations —first from a herbivorous species like the rabbit to an omnivorous species like man, and then from hypercholesteremia or atherosclerosis to myocardial infarctions or sudden cardiac death. Both of these extrapolations are somewhat risky. When done one on top of the other, the chances of reaching meaningful conclusions are slight. It is just not a good research strategy, for scientific peril becomes highly probable. The extrapolations were reasonable in the early stages of research into CHD, but not in the middle or late stages when we are seeking to zero-in on proof of what is happening.

It should not be too difficult to extend the experiments that Sós performed (described in Chapter 8), doing a comparison of yogurt and various milk factors. Some milk factors that should be tested are the proteins casein and lactalbumin, and milk-sugars lactose and galactose. (Sós fed the rats casein.) Different processing of these food factors can have an effect. Thus, partial hydrolysis of casein reduces its cholesterol-elevating properties. [Kritchevsky '85] While experimenting, it would also be worthwhile to determine the effects of other types of milk processing, such as that which produces cottage cheese or buttermilk. Also, it might be worth examining the effects of the dietary lysine to arginine ratio. [Kritchevsky '85] Once more, I wish to emphasize the importance of producing myocardial infarctions or sudden cardiac death in the experimental animals, rather than just elevated blood cholesterol or atherosclerosis.

* * *

With the help of material presented in this book, it is hoped that the astute researcher will be able to put together a unified hypothesis of coronary heart disease, which would be based upon a minimum of assumptions and have considerable elegance. Some judicious experiments on rats will help verify some aspects of it. Additional human epidemiological studies would also be worthwile, if they consider as variables a combination of nutritional factors. More clinical studies, in which individualized nutritional therapy is utilized, must find their way into print.

Assessing Your Nutritional State

As I've mentioned, sooner or later you have to take charge of your own health. The whole question is: **When?** Some will want to do it now; others will want to find a good nutritional practitioner. For serious health problems, you must go to an M. D. Everyone should consider using outside help, at least until they are well on their way to good independent judgment in nutritional matters. This book, or any other book, can't give you all that you need to know. However, I hope that I've given you a good framework within which you can organize nutritional information in your mind. Your first goal will be to get rid of your current health problems, and then prevent new problems from becoming established.

The minimum data that you need for determining your nutritional state are:

1. An analysis of your current diet in terms of the nutrients, to see if you are short-changing yourself in any nutrients. There are two ways to do it: either you can do tedious calculations using food composition tables, or you can use one of the services that will assist with a computer analysis of your diet. You will compare your nutrient intakes to the RDAs. However, you must realize that the diet analysis will be subject to inaccuracies from the fact that foods can vary in nutrient content, and that remembering the foods you've eaten is not very precise.

2. A list of all your health problems, symptoms, signs, and the health history of both you and your ancestors. (If you are blind to your own problems, have your mate help you on this.) Beside each item on this list, you will note (using this and other books, listed below) the deficiencies that are usually associated with each symptom or health problem. You may notice one or several nutrients that appear in your lists over and over again. If these nutrients are the same as the ones that appear somewhat lacking in your diet analysis,

153

then you may be able to solve your problems quickly. Otherwise, you may have a nutrient dependency, needing one or several nutrients far in excess of the RDAs. It is unfortunate that symptoms are not a very reliable guide to extra nutrient needs, since a single symptom could be associated with a variety of health problems, depending upon the individual.

3. It is helpful to study nutritional case histories, from which you may see parallels to your own problems.

4. You are apt to need some hard data on yourself. For this, it is best if you find a physician interested in nutrition, so that you can get proper laboratory tests, which might include nutritional-biochemical tests on blood or urine for vitamins and minerals. Additionally, an assay of the minerals in your hair can be done. Because hair mineral analysis—and its interpretation—is so poorly understood by both the public and the medical profession, I will go into this at length shortly.

I must warn you at this point that no single piece of information will stand alone in making decisions about what you need. No data are totally reliable, including even blood tests that your doctor may make. You must look for patterns, such as a number of pieces of information all pointing in the same direction before you can be certain.

Here are some books (all written in plain English) that can also help you in your efforts:

Dr. Wright's Book of Nutritional Therapy, by Jonathan V. Wright, M. D. (Rodale Press, 1979). Dr. Wright covers case histories of all manner of major and minor diseases. He describes how he handles each case, going into the nutritional therapies and including appropriate nutrient dosages.

Dr. Wright's Guide to Healing With Nutrition, by Jonathan V. Wright, M. D. (Rodale Press, 1984). This sequel to his earlier book also covers case histories, but goes more into allergies, digestive problems, and more recent cases. He also lists organizations that will help you find a good nutritional practitioner.

Dr. Atkins' Nutrition Breakthrough, by Robert C. Atkins, M. D. (Wm. Morrow & Co., 1981). Dr. Atkins is a cardiologist turned nutritional therapist, although he is more widely known for advocating high-protein diets for weight loss.

Nutrition and Vitamin Therapy, by Michael Lesser, M. D. (Grove Press, 1980; Bantam Books, 1981). Dr. Lesser is a Psychiatrist who found that he could help his patients more with nutritional therapy.

Nutrition Almanac, by Nutrition Search, Inc., John D. Kirschmann, Director (McGraw-Hill, 1973, 1975, 1979, and 1984). This book covers a considerable amount of material on the nutrients, nutrient interactions, the various forms of nutritional supplements, the nutrients that help in various ailments, deficiency symptoms, food sources of nutrients, and has tables of the amount of nutrients in standard servings of food.   The book has some flaws: it is a bit too uncritical about the sources of its data, it is inadequate on the trace elements, and it mixes earlier low dosage treatments with later megavitamin treatments.   Early editions had some numerical errors in the food tables.   In spite of all this, it is a useful book.

Super-Nutrition for Healthy Hearts, by Richard A. Passwater, Ph. D. (Dial Press, 1977; Jove/HBJ, 1978).   Dr. Passwater, a biochemist, has written a useful book on heart disease.   However, extensions of knowledge since its publication must be kept in mind.

Trace Elements, Hair Analysis and Nutrition, by Richard A. Passwater, Ph. D., and Elmer M. Cranton, M. D. (Keats, 1983).   This is the most up to date and accurate compilation on the interpretation of hair mineral analysis, and on the trace elements.   The book also includes full references, of use to professionals.

Hair mineral analysis is one of several useful tools for assessing your nutritional state.   However, the test has been getting a bad press the past few years.   The "exposés" in the media would suggest that it is a useless test.   There have been two main problems: Some laboratories doing hair mineral analyses have been using obsolete methods or equipment.   Their results have not been meaningful or reproducible.   The other problem is that the interpretation of the results has been carried too far—that is, all manner of possible diseases have been suggested, based upon the levels of the hair minerals alone.   That is going way too far with the data.   Some laboratories offer computer printouts that tell you what supplements you supposedly need for good health, based only upon the hair minerals.   [Barrett '85]   People are being misled.   Further, some laboratories offer to sell you the supplements they suggest; thus their profit motives are all too apparent.

There is no public access to the better laboratories doing hair mineral analysis.   That is, if you contact them, they will tell you that your hair sample must be submitted through a physician.   Some will give you a list of the physicians in your local area who use the laboratory.   This could help you find a nutritional practitioner.   I've listed (in alphabetical order) the five laboratories that I believe can give you the most reliable measurements of hair minerals.   The cost is modest at all the laboratories.   For convenience, I've included the phone numbers (as of late 1985).

Bio Center Laboratory, Wichita, KS; (316)-684-7784

Davenport Analytical Laboratories, Dallas, TX; (214)-634-1953

Doctor's Data, Inc.; West Chicago, IL; (312)-231-3649

Parmae Laboratories, Dallas, TX; (214)-630-8422

Trace Minerals International, Boulder, CO; (303)-442-1082

(There has been much change in the line-up of hair analysis laboratories in the past year.   Thus, three excellent laboratories are no
longer doing analyses: Trace Analysis Laboratories, MineralLab, and
Graham-Massey Analytical Labs.)
    The fact that needs to be appreciated the most is that the levels
of minerals in the hair often do not reflect the levels of minerals in
the body.   Thus the interpretation of hair minerals is complex and not
fully understood as yet.   Further, the test is not noted for precision.
The results can be rather useful when someone is way out of balance
nutritionally.   Then the skewed patterns of the mineral levels usually
give good clues as to some of the problems.   The hair mineral data
are only to be used along with other nutritional data.   With some
minerals, hair data are more reliable than blood data, because hair
minerals are at a higher concentration than blood minerals, and thus
easier to measure in microscopic amounts.   Also, hair mineral levels
don't depend upon when you had your last meal, as do blood levels.
The test is often useful for determining serious mineral imbalances
and for identifying toxic metal exposures.   Unfortunately, there is
much the test won't do.   Perhaps half the people who have a hair
mineral analysis done won't find anything useful in the results, other
than being able to rule out some possible problems.
    The standard hair sample is from the back of the neck, and
preferably hair that is within an inch or so of the scalp.   Hair that is
further from the scalp, and thus older, can give different results
because of longer exposure to the external environment.   The hair
sample size must be at least 1/2 of a gram and at least a few hundred
hairs, so that normal hair-to-hair variations won't influence the
results.   There are several environmental factors that can change
hair mineral levels.   Two brands of shampoo can affect it: "Selsun
Blue" contains selenium and will raise hair selenium levels; and "Head
& Shoulders" contains zinc and will raise hair zinc levels.   Hair
darkening agents such as "Grecian Formula" contain lead, and raise
hair lead levels sky-high.   The lead is also slowly absorbed and finds

its way into the bones! [Marzulli '78]   If you have been using spray deodorants containing aluminum, it could end up on your hair, giving a false high on the aluminum reading.   If you have a tendency to scratch the back of your head often, any metals that came from your hands can end up being analyzed.   Treatments like bleaching and cold waving alter hair minerals significantly, but permanent waves have less effect.   Since hair grows an inch every few months, it is best to wait at least a few months after any of these products or treatments have been used before taking a hair sample for mineral analysis. Alternatively, pubic hair can be used, but the "normal" mineral levels are far different, perhaps partly because pubic hair grows much more slowly.   Note that hair mineral levels are also influenced somewhat by age, sex and grey hair.

There is no need to wash your hair before the sample is taken, as the laboratory will wash your hair sample with detergents or solvents far stronger than you could ever use.   After washing, the sample is digested and cooked in acid to get rid of all hair protein.   There are several different ways of measuring the remaining metals.   Four of the laboratories I've listed use a method called "atomic absorption spectroscopy."   The other laboratory (Doctor's Data, Inc.) uses a method called "vacuum ICP" (inductively coupled plasma).   Each method has its advantages, but I feel the former has a slight edge when it comes to accuracy and repeatability of measurements.

Normal variation in results when the test is repeated is perhaps 25%.   Many of the above mentioned additional causes of variation may influence the results another 25 to 50% or more.   Thus, uncontrolled factors may change hair mineral levels by a factor of two or so.   This only tells us not to try to interpret modest variations from the normal ranges.   Hair mineral analysis can be most useful when variations are seen that are 5 to 10 times (or more) off the normal levels.

If the results come out highly abnormal, an immediate retest can be requested of the laboratory.   Retests can also be done a year later to check progress of the nutritional therapy.   Whenever results come out fairly normal, there is no reason to repeat the test for many years, at least.

Most hair analysis laboratories give readings on from fifteen to thirty different minerals and trace elements.   The quality control methods used by the laboratory are more important than having readings on a large number of minerals.   At present, we are not able to interpret more than a dozen nutritional minerals and half a dozen toxic minerals, at most.   Measurement of some nutritional minerals is only of limited usefulness, possibly in rare circumstances.   The nutritional minerals that are worth getting readings on include: calcium, magnesium, sodium, potassium, iron, copper, zinc, chromium, manganese, selenium, nickel and vanadium. It is possible to detect toxic levels of lead, mercury, cadmium, arsenic, or aluminum.

The mineral levels are usually expressed in the units "mg%," which stands for milligrams percent, and means the number of milligrams of an element in 100 grams of hair. Scientists are more likely to be using "ppm," which is parts per million, or micrograms of the element in a gram of hair. If you have to convert, just remember that 1 mg% equals 10 ppm, or that you multiply the numbers by 10 when you convert readings from mg% to ppm.

Now let us consider what the hair mineral levels can tell us. Note that for the nutritional minerals, **low** means low relative to the normal range, and **high** means high relative to the normal range. You'll find that the laboratories differ in their "normal" ranges, caused mainly by different washing and measuring procedures. For the toxic minerals, there are given ideally low levels, and the toxic levels.

Calcium, magnesium, sodium and potassium: The hair levels of these four electrolyte minerals can not be relied upon to give a good indication of nutritional status.

With calcium and magnesium, low hair levels usually suggest inadequate intake. But high hair levels of both can also indicate inadequate intake. The mechanism is uncertain, but a high hair calcium may mean that calcium is coming out of the bones and being deposited in the soft tissues (which is certainly an adverse effect), and that the magnesium in the hair is just following calcium. In this situation of high hair calcium and magnesium, there can well be low levels of magnesium in most of the body, especially in the heart muscle cells. On the other hand, if one has been taking excessive calcium supplementation, the hair calcium will be high, with a low hair magnesium. The normal ratio of hair calcium to hair magnesium is about 6 to 1. Sometimes an abnormal ratio is meaningful.

Frequently, hair levels of lead or aluminum can give clues as to the body's calcium and magnesium status.   Ideally, hair lead level is only 0.1 mg%, but if it is elevated five times or more above that, it is possible the individual has an inadequate calcium intake.   The ideally low hair aluminum level is about 0.2 mg%, but if it is up around 1 mg% or more, there is a good chance that the individual has had too low a magnesium intake.

Sodium and potassium hair levels are frequently not meaningful. Sometimes a high hair sodium indicates too high a dietary intake of sodium. Other times a high hair sodium will be seen in hypoglycemics, usually with a low chromium level. The normal ratio of sodium to potassium in the hair is about 2 to 1, but it can vary widely. Occasionally, a reversed ratio, 1 to 2 (i. e., sodium to potassium of less than 0.5), tells the nutritional therapist to look for signs of celiac disease (which results from an intolerance to wheat gluten).

I found a highly unique pattern between calcium, potassium and sodium that could warn of the danger of sudden cardiac death. Three out of eight middle-aged men (ages 39 to 60) who had died of sudden cardiac death showed a sky-high hair potassium level, with calcium level average or above, and sodium level above average. (Examining the hair mineral patterns of many hundreds of people, I've noticed that, if potassium is high, calcium will be found low; or if calcium is high, potassium will be found low. That is my reason for calling the pattern found in sudden cardiac death "unique.") The likely danger zone for sudden cardiac death is when the product of hair calcium and hair potassium reaches about 2000 or more (using units of mg%). I came across one live male whose hair levels were close to this zone, and he happened to show several signs of severe atherosclerosis. With nutritional therapy, hair mineral levels gradually returned to normal. He then appeared to be in much better health. [However, the above formula for warning of sudden cardiac death may only work with the results from some laboratories. The readings on potassium can vary tremendously between different laboratories, because of differences in wash procedures. These particular analyses were carried out at the Trace Analysis Laboratory, noted for the best repeatability in results, but which no longer does hair mineral analysis. Further research is needed to determine the reliability of this early warning indicator.]

Iron: Hair iron levels are relatively inadequate for determining body iron status. Extremes, either high or low, can be suggestive of excessive or inadequate intakes. The best measure of body iron status is blood serum ferritin, which is much better than either blood hemoglobin or hair iron.

Copper: Hair copper gives a good measure of body status, in some people at least. A low level suggests deficiency. A high level usually suggests excess copper in the body, but occasionally indicates a low level in the body. Symptoms of zinc deficiency are the most reliable sign of copper excess, because excess copper can interfere with zinc enzymes in the body. If you swim in a pool frequently, it may elevate the copper in your hair.

Zinc: Hair zinc is a more reliable indicator of body zinc status than blood zinc, but it is not much better. Both are relatively uncertain as indicators. White spots on the fingernails are the one sure sign of zinc deficiency. But many people with inadequate zinc status don't show white spots. A low hair zinc suggests zinc deficiency. A high hair zinc also suggests deficiency, unless the person has been supplementing excessive quantities of zinc for a substantial period of time.

The normal ratio of zinc to copper in the hair is about 8 to 1. Sometimes this ratio is helpful in determining whether to emphasize supplementation of zinc, or of copper.

Manganese: Americans have much lower manganese levels in their hair than people in the underdeveloped countries, most likely because our methods of agriculture short our foods. It is worthwhile supplementing with manganese when hair manganese is way below normal. High hair manganese is seen in some cases of magnesium deficiency, but can also be seen in those who have an industrial exposure to manganese.

Chromium: Low hair chromium levels are suggestive of problems with blood sugar regulation. But a sky-high hair chromium can also be an indication of chromium deficiency (unless the person has been exposed to industrial chromates). The best absorbed chromium supplement is GTF-chromium, as previously mentioned.

Selenium: Hair analysis laboratories are getting better at measuring selenium with reasonable accuracy. You wouldn't want to be misled by a false reading. With a truly low hair selenium level, supplementation is advisable. Without a good measurement, it is best to restrict yourself to modest supplementation, of the order of 100 micrograms, because excess selenium is toxic.

In the previous nutritional minerals, you want to find them somewhere near the normal range, but the following **toxic minerals** you would hope to find in low concentrations:

Lead: The ideally low level of hair lead is about 0.1 mg%. With levels above 0.5 mg%, you might be wise to increase your intake of the nutritional minerals that block lead absorption: calcium, magnesium, zinc, iron and selenium. Symptoms of lead toxicity begin around 3.0 mg%, but by the time you have that level, you've already accumulated substantial lead in your bones. Before becoming panicky about a high hair lead level, do a retest using pubic hair.   Head hair is easily contaminated with lead, without any in the body.   The most likely contamination comes from using hair-darkening agents.

Aluminum: The ideally low hair aluminum level is about 0.2 mg%.   A level above 1.0 mg% may suggest a magnesium deficiency.   Toxicity begins around 3.0 mg%, but many people with levels higher than that will show no symptoms.   The symptoms only occur if the aluminum gets into your brain.   Fortunately, the brain has a good barrier against aluminum.

Cadmium: The ideally low hair cadmium level is about 0.03 mg% or so.   However, many laboratories can't measure cadmium at this low a level.   Because cadmium accumulates in the kidney cortex, and starts doing its damage there, confirmed evidence of elevated hair cadmium should be dealt with promptly through supplementation with zinc, copper, iron, selenium and vitamin C.

Mercury: The ideally low level of hair mercury is 0.01 mg% or less. Levels up to 0.3 mg% may be considered acceptable, but it is best to work toward lowering any elevated mercury level with selenium supplementation.   Note that some brands of shampoo contain mercury as a preservative.   This could elevate hair mercury.

Arsenic: Arsenic levels up to about 0.15 mg% can be considered as harmless.

Bismuth: An excess of bismuth can cause mental and neuromuscular problems.   Bismuth is used in certain medicines and cosmetics.   Not many hair analysis laboratories can detect it.

If you are planning to do-it-yourself, be cautious.   An excess of self-confidence in your abilities is not wise, at any level of knowledge.   With possibly serious health problems, you must see an M. D.

Reference Notes

No attempt has been made to support all of my statements with references, since that would have entailed writing the book in a different style and citing many thousands of papers, perhaps adding more confusion than enlightenment. Many of the references have been selected to help researchers follow (and check) my reasoning on the diet/CHD story. I have tried to cite the latest review paper in any area. I have also cited important earlier work that seems to have been forgotten, or was never noticed because of being published in less widely circulated medical journals. Most of the references are specific, but a few are inserted for good general background on a topic. Those desiring further references on general nutritional therapy will find them in abundance in other books on the subject.

Ames, Bruce N.: The detection of environmental mutagens and potential carcinogens. Cancer 53(10): 2034-2040 (15 May **1984**)

Ames, Bruce N.: Identifying environmental chemicals causing mutations and cancer. Science 204: 587-593 (11 May **1979**)

Altura, B. M.: Sudden-death ischemic heart disease and dietary magnesium intake: Is the target site coronary vascular smooth muscle? Medical Hypotheses 5: 843-848 (**1979**) [The Alturas have extended their work to the microcirculation in the rest of the body, giving more complete mechanisms of action. See Science for 23 Mar 1984, pages 1315-1317.]

Altura, B. T.: Type-A behavior and coronary vasospasm: A possible role of hypomagnesemia. Medical Hypotheses 6: 753-757 (**1980**)

Anderson, Terence W., et al: Magnesium, water hardness, and heart disease. Pages 565-571 in Magnesium in Health and Disease, ed. by Cantin and Seelig (Spectrum **1980**)

Anderson, Terence W.: A new view of heart disease. New Scientist 77: 374-376 (9 Feb **1978**)

Anderson, Terence W., et al: Ischemic heart disease, water hardness and myocardial magnesium. Can. Med. Assoc. J. 113: 199-203 (9 Aug 1975)

Anderson, Terence W.: The changing pattern of ischemic heart disease. Can. Med. Assoc. J. 108: 1500-1504 (23 Jun 1973)

Annand, J. C.: Further evidence in the case against heated milk protein. Atherosclerosis 15: 129-133 (1972). For earlier work, see: Atherosclerosis 13: 137-139 (1971), and J. Atherosclerosis Research 7: 797-801 (1967)

Arntzenius, Alexander C., et al: Diet, lipoproteins, and the progression of coronary atherosclerosis. New England J. of Med. 312: 805-811 (28 Mar 1985)

Barrett, Stephen: Commercial hair analysis; science or scam? JAMA 254(8): 1041-1045 (23/30 Aug 1985)

Beamish, Robert E.: Stress and Heart Disease. (Proc. of the Int'l. Symposium on Stress and Heart Disease, held in Winnipeg, 26-29 Jun 1984) Edited by Robert E. Beamish, Pawan K. Singal, and Naranjan S. Dhalla. (Martinus Nijhoff Publ. 1985)

Behr, G., and P. Burton: Heart-muscle magnesium. The Lancet, 25 Aug 1973, p. 450

Benet, Sula: How to Live to be 100. (Dial Press 1976) She quotes, from Russian medical statistics, the 1964 disease incidence figures for Dagestan, per 100,000 people. The figures are for the mountains, the foothills, and the plains, respectively:

heart attacks:	0.17	0.2	1.2
strokes:	4.1	7.3	46.8
hypertension:	13.0	38.8	80.6

[The U. S. figure for heart attacks is well over 500.]

Bigg, Roland: Magnesium: The neglected cation. Med. J. Australia 2(6): 340-341 (20 Sep 1980)

Biss, Kurt, et al: Some unique biological characteristics of the Masai of East Africa. New Engl. J. Med. 284: 694-699 (1 Apr 1971)

Bordia, A. K.: Effect of vitamin C on blood lipids, fibrinolytic activity, platelet adhesiveness in patients with coronary artery disease. Atherosclerosis 35: 181-187 (Jan-Apr 1980)

Briggs, R. D., et al: Myocardial infarction in patients treated with Sippy and other high milk diets: an autopsy study of 15 hospitals in the U. S. A. and Great Britain. Circ. 21: 538-542 (Apr **1960**)

Brin, Myron: Red cell transketolase as an indicator of nutritional deficiency. Am. J. Clin. Nutr. 33: 169-171 (Feb **1980**)

Brown, J. O., et al: Nutritional and epidemiological features related to heart disease. Wld. Rev. Nutr. Dietet. 12: 1-42 (**1970**)

Browne, S. E.: Magnesium and cardiovascular disease. (Letter) Brit. Med. J. for 13 July **1963**, p. 118

Burch, G. E., and T. D. Giles: The importance of magnesium deficiency in cardiovascular disease. Am. Heart J. 94:649-657 (Nov **1977**)

Bushnell, Philip J., and Hector F. DeLuca: Lactose facilitates the intestinal absorption of Pb in weanling rats. Science 211: 61-63 (2 Jan **1981**)

Calabrese, Edward J.: Nutrition and Environmental Health (The Influence of Nutritional Status on Pollutant Toxicity and Carcinogenicity) Volume 1, **1980.** Volume 2, **1981.**

Cantin, Marc: Magnesium in Health and Disease, ed. by Marc Cantin and Mildred S. Seelig. Proceedings of the Second International Symposium on Magnesium, in Montreal, May 30-June 1, 1976 (Spectrum **1980**)

Chipperfield, Barbara, and J. R. Chipperfield: Differences in metal content of the heart muscle in death from ischemic heart disease. Am. Heart J. 95(6): 732-737 (Jun **1978**)

Chipperfield, Barbara, et al: Magnesium and potassium content of normal heart muscle in areas of hard and soft water. The Lancet, 17 Jan. **1976**, pp. 121-122. [Note well that neither the hard nor the soft water contains significant magnesium, according to a later paper by Chipperfield (Lancet, 6 Oct 1979, p. 710), and thus their work in no way contradicts Anderson's work that found water hard with magnesium to be protective in heart disease.]

Chutkow, J. G.: The neurophysiologic function of Mg: effects of Mg excess and deficit. Pages 713-752 in Magnesium in Health and Disease, ed. by Marc Cantin and Mildred S. Seelig. (Spectrum **1980**)

Cohen, Leon, and Ruth Kitzes: Magnesium sulfate and digitalis-toxic arrhythmias. JAMA 249(20):2808-2810 (27 May **1983**) [Used the lymphocyte-magnesium test for heart muscle-Mg]

Connor, William E., et al: The plasma lipids, lipoproteins, and diet of the Tarahumara Indians of Mexico. AJCN 31: 1131-1142 (Jul **1978**) [Note earlier papers quoted on the lack of heart disease, such as paper by D. Groom in Am. Heart J. 81: 304, 1971.]

Crapo, Phyllis: The glycemic index. Nutrition Today, Mar/Apr **1984**, p. 6ff

Davies, I. J. T.: The Clinical Significance of the Essential Biological Metals. (Charles C. Thomas **1972**)

Davis, W. H., and F. Ziady: The effect of oral magnesium chloride on the QTc and QUc intervals in the electrocardiogram. So. Afr. Med. J., 15 April **1978**, pp. 591-593.

Day, José, et al: Anthropometric, physiological and biochemical differences between urban and rural Masai. Atherosclerosis 23: 357-361 (**1976**)

Douglas, Loudon M.: The Bacillus of Long Life. G. P. Putnam's Sons **1911**

Dyckner, Thomas, and Per Ola Wester: Relation between potassium, magnesium, and cardiac arrhythmias. Pages 163-169 in Acta Medica Scand. Suppl. 647 (**1981**)

Dyckner, Thomas: Serum magnesium in acute myocardial infarction (relation to arrhythmias). Acta Med. Scand. 207: 59-66 (**1980**)

Ebel, H., and T. Gunther: Magnesium metabolism: a review. J. Clin. Chem. Clin. Biochem. 18(5): 257-270 (May **1980**)

Elwood, P. C., et al: Magnesium and calcium in the myocardium: cause of death and area difference. The Lancet, 4 Oct **1980**, pp. 720-722

Enloe, Cortez F., Jr.: Coronary disease prevention should be individualized. Nutrition Today, Mar/Apr **1984**, pp.12-14. For his further editorial comments, see the Jan/Feb 1985 issue, page 10.

Flink, Edmund B.: Magnesium deficiency, etiology and clinical spectrum. Pages 125-137 in Acta Medica Scandinavica, Suppl. 647 (**1981**)

Flink, Edmund B.: Nutritional aspects of magnesium metabolism. Western J. of Medicine 133: 304-312 (Oct **1980**)

Flink, Edmund B., et al: Relationship of free fatty acids and magnesium in ethanol withdrawal in dogs. Metabolism 28: 858-865 (Aug **1979**)

Flink, Edmund B.: Magnesium deficiency as a cause of serious arrhythmias. (Letter) Arch. Intern. Med. 138: 825 (May **1978**)

Follis, Richard H., Jr.: The effects of nutritional deficiency on the heart: A review. AJCN 4(2): 107-116 (Mar/Apr **1956**)

Fouty, Robert A.: Liquid protein diet magnesium deficiency and cardiac arrest. (Letter) JAMA 240(24): 2632 (8 Dec **1978**)

Friedman, Meyer: (Papers on type A behavior, **1984-1980**) See Amer. Heart J. 108(2): 237-248 (Aug 1984); JAMA 252(11): 1385-1393 (21 Sep 1984); Circ. 66(1): 83-92 (1982); The Sciences, Feb 1980, pages 10, 11, and 28.

Friend, Berta, Louise Page, and Ruth Marston: Food Consumption Patterns in the U. S. A., 1909-1976. Pages 489-522 in Nutrition, Lipids and Coronary Heart Disease, ed. by Robert I. Levy, et al. (Ravens Press **1979**)

Friend, Berta: Nutrients in the United States food supply. Am. J. Clin. Nutr. 20: 907-914 (Aug **1967**)

Geiderman, Joel M., et al: Magnesium—the forgotten electrolyte. JACEP 8: 204-208 (May **1979**)

Ghani, M. Farooq, and M. Rabah: Effect of magnesium chloride on electrical stability of the heart. Am. Heart J. 94: 600-602 (Nov **1977**)

Gibney, M. J., and P. G. Burstyn: Milk, serum cholesterol, and the Maasai. Atherosclerosis 35: 339-343 **(1980)**

Ginter, Emil: Decline of coronary mortality in the U. S. and vitamin C. (Letter) Am. J. Clin. Nutr. 32(3): 511-512 **(1979)**

Glomset, John A.: Fish, fatty acids, and human health. (Editorial) New England J. of Medicine 312(19): 1253-1254 (9 May **1985**) [See also three other papers on omega-3 oil in this issue.]

Graber, Thomas W., et al: Magnesium: physiology, clinical disorders, and therapy. Ann. Emerg. Med. 10: 49-57 (Jan **1981**)

Guberan, E.: Surprising decline of cardiovascular mortality in Switzerland: 1951-1976. J. of Epidemiology and Community Health 33: 114-120 (**1979**)

Guerci, A.: Sudden death—Medical Staff Conference. Western J. of Med. 133: 313-320 (Oct **1980**)

Gunther, T., et al: Biochemical mechanisms in magnesium deficiency. Pages 57-65 in Magnesium in Health and Disease, ed. by Marc Cantin and Mildred S. Seelig. (Spectrum **1980**)

Hartroft, W. Stanley, et al: Experimental production of coronary atherosclerosis. Am. J. Cardiol. 9: 355-364 (Mar **1962**)

Ho, K-J., et al: The Masai of East Africa: Some unique biological characteristics. Arch. Pathol. 91: 387-410 (**1971**)

Hoffer, Abram: Nutrition and behavior. Pages 222-251 in Medical Applications of Clinical Nutrition, ed. by Jeffrey Bland (Keats **1983**)

Holtmeier, H. J., and M. Kuhn: Problems of nutritional intake of calcium and magnesium and their possible influence on coronary disease. Pages 671-677 in Magnesium in Health and Disease, ed. by Marc Cantin and Mildred S. Seelig. (Spectrum **1980**)

Hubbard, Jeffrey D., et al: Nathan Pritikin's heart. New England J. of Med. 313: 52 (4 Jul **1985**)

Isaacs, James P., et al: Trace metals, vitamins, and hormones in long-term treatment of coronary atherosclerotic heart disease. Pages 313-327 in Trace Substances in Environmental Health, Volume 5, ed. by Delbert D. Hemphill. (Proc. of the Univ. of Missouri's Fifth Annual Conf. on T. S. in E. H., **1971**). [In this study, 25 cases were followed for 10 years. In a later study, 100 additional cases were taken on. I have been unable to successfully track down the latest results.]

Iseri, Lloyd T, et al: Magnesium deficiency and cardiac disorders. Am. J. Med. 58: 837-846 (June **1975**)

Janke, J., et al: Prevention of myocardial Ca overload and necrotization by Mg and K salts or acidosis. Pages 33-42 in Recent Advances in Studies in Cardiac Structure and Metabolism, Volume 6, ed. by Albrecht Fleckenstein and George Rona. (University Park Press **1975**)

Jenkins, David J. A., et al: The Glycaemic response to carbohydrate foods. Lancet, 18 Aug **1984**, pp. 388-391

Johnson, Carl J., et al: Myocardial tissue concentrations of magnesium and potassium in men dying suddenly from ischemic heart disease. Am. J. Clin. Nutr. 32: 967-970 (May **1979**)

Judd, Joseph T., June L. Kelsay, and Walter Mertz: Potential risks from low-fat diets. Seminars in Oncology 10(3): 273-280 (Sep **1983**)

Kannel, William B., and Joseph Stokes III: Epidemiology of coronary artery disease. Pages 63-88 in Diagnosis and Therapy of Coronary Artery Disease (Second edition), edited by Peter F. Cohn (Martinus Nijhoff Publishing **1985**)

Kaplan, Norman M.: Non-drug treatment of hypertension. Ann. Int. Med. 102(3): 359-373 (Mar **1985**)

Kare, Morley R.: The Chemical Senses and Nutrition, ed. by Morley R. Kare and Owen Maller. Academic Press **1977**

Karppanen, H., et al: Minerals, coronary heart disease and sudden coronary death. Adv. Cardiol. 25: 9-24 (**1978**)

Katholi, Richard E., et al: Dual dependence on both Ca^{2+} and Mg^{2+} for electrical stability in cells of canine false tendon. J. of Molecular and Cellular Cardiology **1979**, p. 435-445.

Kimura, Noboru: Changing patterns of CHD, stroke, and nutrient intakes in Japan. Preventive Medicine 12(1): 222-227 (Jan **1983**)

Kiyosawa, Haruo, et al: Effect of skim milk and yogurt on serum lipids and development of sudanophilic lesions in cholesterol-fed rabbits. Am. J. Clin. Nutr. 40: 479-484 (Sep **1984**)

Klevay, Leslie M.: Mg, Ca, Cu and Zn in meals. (Correlations related to the epidemiology of ischemic heart disease.) Biological Trace Element Research 4: 95-104 (Jun/Sep **1982**)

Klevay, Leslie M.: Interactions of copper and zinc in cardiovascular disease. Annals of the New York Academy of Sciences, Volume 355, pages 140-151 (**1980**)

Kolata, Gina: Heart panel's conclusions questioned. Science 227: 40-41 (4 Jan **1985**)

Kritchevsky, David: How does plant protein reduce serum cholesterol levels? Nutrition & The M. D. 11(6): 3 (Jun **1985**)

Kummerow, Fred A.: Nutrition imbalance and angiotoxins as dietary risk factors in coronary heart disease. AJCN 32: 58-83 (**1979**)

Kummerow, Fred A., et al: Additive risk factors in atherosclerosis.
    Am. J. Clin. Nutr. 29: 579-584 (May **1976**)

Kushi, Lawrence H., et al.:   Diet and 20-year mortality from
    coronary heart disease.   New England J. of Medicine 312(13):
    811-818 (28 Mar **1985**)

Lehr, D., et al: Possible role of magnesium loss in the pathogenesis
    of myocardial fiber necrosis.   Pages 95-109 in Recent Advan-
    ces in Studies on Cardiac Structure and Metabolism, Volume 6,
    ed. by Albrecht Fleckenstein and George Rona.   (University
    Park **1975**)

Leibovitz, Brian: Carnitine. The Vitamin B_T Phenomenon.   (Dell
    1984)

Linden, Victor: Correlation of vitamin D intake to ischemic heart
    disease, hypercholesterolemia, and renal calcinosis.   Pages 23-
    42 in Nutritional Imbalances in Infant and Adult Disease, edited
    by Mildred Seelig.   (Spectrum **1977**) [Note that Torstein Vik
    et al (Brit. Med. J., 21 July 1979, p. 176) argued against Linden's
    conclusions upon finding normal vitamin D levels in blood serum
    of those who had died of CHD.   However, because excessive
    vitamin D tends to accumulate in muscle and adipose tissue
    rather than in blood serum (E. B. Mawer et al, Clin. Sci. 43: 413,
    1972), Vik's results on blood serum are not pertinent.]

LRC, Lipid Research Clinics Coronary Primary Prevention Trials
    Results.   JAMA 251: 351ff (20 Jan **1984**).   [Comments con-
    cerning the results will be found in Nutrition Today 1984.
    Several researchers criticized the statistical methods used to
    analyze the data, and suggested that the LRC-CPPT results
    were not statistically significant.   See also Kolata 1985.]

Loeb, Henry S., et al: Paroxysmal ventricular fibrillation in two
    patients with hypomagnesemia.   Circ. 37: 210-215 **(1968)**

Lowenstein, F. W.:   Epidemiological investigations in relation to diet
    in groups who show little atherosclerosis and are almost free of
    CHD.   Am. J. Clin. Nutr. 15: 175-186 (Sep **1964**)

Lown, Bernard: Sudden cardiac death: the major challenge con-
    fronting contemporary cardiology.   Am. J. Cardiol. 43: 313-328
    (Feb **1979**)

Lown, Bernard, et al: Neural and psychologic mechanisms and the
    problem of sudden cardiac death.   Am. J. Cardiol. 39: 890-902
    (26 May **1977**)

Mahaffey, Kathryn R.:   Nutrient-Pb interactions.   Pages 425-460 in Lead Toxicity, ed. by R. L. Singhal and J. A. Thomas. (Urban and Schwarzenberg **1980**)   [Note additionally that Pb causes mitochondrial swelling (p. 150, op cit), certainly a phenomenon adverse to normal heart metabolism.]

Malkiel-Shapiro, B., and I. Bersohn: Magnesium sulphate in coronary thrombosis.   (Notes and comments)   Brit. Med. J. for 23 Jan **1960,** p. 292.

Mann, George V.:   A factor in yogurt which lowers cholesteremia in man.   Atherosclerosis 26: 335-340 **(1977)**

Mann, George V., et al: Atherosclerosis in the Masai.   Am. J. Epidemiology 95: 26-37 **(1972)**

Mann, George V., et al: Cardiovascular disease in the Masai.   J. Atherosclerosis Research 4: 289-312 **(1964)**

Marier, J. R.:   The role of Mg in the cardio-protective effect of hard water.   (in French)   Can. Med. Nutr. 16(1): 23-29 **(1980)**

Marier, J. R., Luciano Neri, and Terence W. Anderson: Water hardness, Human Health, and the Importance of Magnesium.   Canadian Nat'l. Res. Council, Publication 17581.   Ottawa **1979**

Marston, Ruth M., and Susan O. Welsh: Nutrient content of the national food supply.   Nat'l Food Rev., Winter **1981,** pp. 19-22

Martin, Wayne: The beri-beri analogy to myocardial infarction. Medical Hypotheses 10: 185-198 (Feb **1983**)

Marzulli, F. N., et al: Uptake of systemic Pb, hair as a test tissue. Curr. Probl. Dermatol. 7: 196-204 **(1978)**

Maugh, Thomas H, II: Hair: a diagnostic tool to complement blood serum and urine.   Science 202: 1271-1274 (22 Dec **1978**)

McGee, Charles T.:   How to Survive Modern Technology.   (Ecology Press **1979**)

Mertz, Walter: Food and nutrients.   J. Amer. Dietetic Assoc. 84(7): 769-770 (Jul **1984**)

Mertz, Walter: (Various papers on the trace elements, **1984-1980**) See the three part series in Nutrition Today for Jan/Feb 1984 (p. 22ff), Sep/Oct 1983 (p. 26ff), Mar/Apr 1983 (p. 6ff).   Also see Science 213: 1332-1338 (18 Sep 1981) and J. Am. Dietetic Assoc. 77: 258-263 (Sep 1980)

Miller, D. R., and K. C. Hayes: Vitamin excess and toxicity.   Pages 81-133 in Nutritional Toxicology, Volume 1, ed. by John N. Hathcock. (Academic Press **1982**)

Mordes, J. P., and W. Wacker: Excess magnesium.   Pharmacol. Rev. 29(4): 273-300 (Dec **1977**)

Neal, John B., and Marybelle Neal: Effect of hard water and $MgSO_4$ on rabbit atherosclerosis.   Archives of Pathology 73: 400-403 (May **1962**)

Neri, L. C., and J. R. Marier: Epidemiology of sudden cardiac death: Minerals and the "water story".   Pages 81-96 in Nutrition and Heart Disease (Monographs of the Amer. College of Nutrition, vol. 5), ed. by H. Naito.   (Spectrum **1982**)

Neri, Luciano C., and Helen L. Johansen: Water Hardness and cardiovascular mortality.   Annals of the New York Academy of Sciences, Volume 304, pages 203-221.   (**1978**)

Nutrition Today: Note that controversies over nutrition and heart disease have been well covered, with comments by experts from around the world.   See especially the issues of Mar/Apr, Sep/Oct, Nov/Dec **1984**, and May/Jun, Jul/Aug, Sep/Oct **1980**.

Oliver, Michael F.:   (Comments on the LRC-CPPT findings)   See p. 27 of Nutrition Today, Sep/Oct **1984**

Oliver, Michael F.:   Should we not forget about mass control of coronary risk factors?   Lancet, 2 July **1983**, pp. 37-38

Olsen, Elsie A., et al: Topical minoxidil in early male pattern baldness.   J. of Amer. Acad. of Dermatology 13(2): 185-192 (Aug **1985**)

Opie, Lionel H.:   Cardiac metabolism: Catecholamines, calcium, cyclic AMP, and substrates.   Pages 3-20 in Advances in Myocardiology, Volume 1, ed. by M. Tajuddin et al.   (University Park **1980**)

Oster, Kurt A., et al: The XO Factor.   (Park City Press **1983**)

Oster, Kurt A.:   Atherosclerosis: conjectures, data and facts. Nutrition Today, Nov/Dec **1981**, p. 28-29.

Oster, Kurt A.:   Cholesterol and CHD.   Circulation 60(2): 463-464 (August **1979**) [A letter, with reply by Osmo Turpeinen.]

Passwater, Richard A., and Elmer M. Cranton: Trace Elements, Hair Analysis and Nutrition. (Keats **1983**)

Peng, Shi-Kaung, and C. Bruce Taylor: Cholesterol autoxidation, health and arteriosclerosis. World Rev. Nutr. Dietet. 44: 117-154 (**1984**)

Pfeiffer, Carl C.: Zinc and Other Micro-Nutrients. (Keats **1978**)

Pfeiffer, Carl C.: Mental and Elemental Nutrients. (Keats **1975**)

Pihl, Robert O.: Hair element content in learning disabled children. Science 198: 204-206 (14 Oct **1977**)

Pinckney, Edward R., and Cathey Pinckney: The Cholesterol Controversy. (Sherbourne **1973**)

Polimeni, Phillip I., and Ernest Page: Magnesium in heart muscle. Circulation Research 33: 367-374 (Oct **1973**)

Popham, Robert E., et al: Variation in mortality from ischemic heart disease in relation to alcohol and milk consumption. Medical Hypotheses 12: 321-329 (Dec **1983**)

Raab, W.: Myocardial electrolyte derangement: Crucial feature of pluricausal, so-called coronary, heart disease. Annals of the New York Academy of Sciences, volume 147, pp. 629-686 (**1969**)

Rabkin, Simon W., et al: Chronobiology of sudden cardiac death in men. JAMA 244(12): 1357-1358 (19 Sep **1980**)

Reddy, Bandaru S., et al: Fecal constituents of a high-risk North American and a low-risk Finnish population for the development of large bowel cancer. Cancer Letters 4: 217-222 (Apr **1978**)

Robinson, Miles H.: On sugar and white flour: The dangerous twins! Pages 24-30 in A Physician's Handbook on Orthomolecular Medicine, ed. by Roger J. Williams and Dwight K. Kalita. (Pergamon **1977**)

Roe, Daphne A.: Nutrient and drug interactions. Nutrition Rev. 42(4): 141-154 (Apr **1984**)

Rose, G. A.: Corn oil in treatment of ischaemic heart disease. Brit. Med. J. 5449: 1531-1533 (12 Jun **1965**)

Rudin, Donald O.: The dominant diseases of modernized societies as omega-3 EFA deficiency syndrome: substrate beri-beri. Medical Hypotheses 8: 17-47 (Jan **1982**)

Schachne, Jay S., et al: Coronary artery spasm and myocardial infarction associated with cocaine use.   New England J. of Med. 310: 1665-1666 (21 Jun **1984**)

Schauss, Alexander G.:   Diet, Crime and Delinquency.   (Parker House **1980**)

Schoenthaler, Stephen J.:   Institutional nutritional policies and criminal behavior.   Nutrition Today 20(3): 16-24 (May/Jun **1985**)

Schroeder, Henry A., et al: Essential metals in man: magnesium.   J. Chron. Dis. 21: 815-841 (**1969**)

Seelig, Mildred S.:   Magnesium Deficiency in the Pathogenesis of Disease (Early Roots of Cardiovascular, Skeletal, and Renal Abnormalities)   Plenum **1980**

Seelig, Mildred S., and H. Alexander Heggtveit: Magnesium inter-relationships in ischemic heart disease: a review.   Am. J. Clin. Nutr. 27: 59-79 (Jan **1974**)

Seely, Stephen: Diet and cerebrovascular disease: Search for linkages.   Medical Hypotheses 9: 509-515 (**1982**)

Seely, Stephen: Diet and coronary disease: a survey of mortality rates and food consumption statistics of 24 countries.   Medical Hypotheses 7: 907-918 (July **1981**) [As pointed out by R. J. Pearce (Med. Hypotheses 14(3): 259-260, Jul 1984), Seely's category "milk proteins" should actually be called milk-solids-non-fat.   This fraction contains lactose, protein, ash, vitamins, and cofactors (in descending order of concentration).   During fermentation, most of the lactose is converted to lactic acid, the proteins are coagulated, and many of the dissolved nutrients are removed (in cheese making).   The point is, the problem with milk is not necessarily in the protein (unless its coagulation somehow removes the problem), but could well be in the lactose portion.]

Segall, Jeffrey J.: Hypothesis: Is lactose a dietary risk factor for ischaemic heart disease?   International J. of Epidemiology 9(3): 271-276 (**1980**)

Segall, Jeffrey J.:   (Letter about wine drinkers, milk drinkers, and CHD) Lancet 1 (8129):1294 (16 June **1979**)

Segall, Jeffrey J.: Is milk a coronary health hazard?   Brit. J. of Preventive and Social Medicine 31: 81-85 (**1977**)

Shamberger, Raymond J.:   Trace metals in health and disease.
Pages 241-275 in Nutritional Elements and Clinical Biochemistry, ed. by Marge A. Brewster and Herbert K. Naito (Plenum
1980).

Sharrett, Richey A.:   The role of chemical constituents of drinking
water in cardiovascular disease.   Pages 69-81 in Geochemistry
of Water in Relation to Cardiovascular Disease, by a U. S.
National Committee for Geochemistry. (National Academy of
Sciences **1979**).   [On page 78, it says that the work from
England (Chipperfield 1976) apparently contradicts the work
from Ontario (Anderson 1975) concerning hard water.   Unfortunately, the Committee didn't know that English water, hard or
soft, contains negligible magnesium (of the order of 2 to 5 ppm).
The Committee was unable to reach favorable conclusions on
the heart-protective role of magnesium in hard water, because
they had inadequate facts on hand.]

Shils, Maurice E.:   Magnesium.   Pages 247-258 in Nutrition Review's
Present Knowledge in Nutrition, fourth edition, ed. by D. Mark
Hegsted et al.   (The Nutrition Foundation **1976**)

Shute, Wilfred E.:   Tailoring the dose.   Pages 67-70 in Physician's
Handbook on Orthomolecular Medicine, ed. by Roger J. Williams
and Dwight K. Kalita (Pergamon Press **1977**)

Sinclair, Hugh M.:   See p. 70 in Nutrition and Killer Diseases, ed. by
John Rose (Noyes Publ. **1982**)

Singh, Narayani P., et al: Intake of magnesium and toxicity of lead:
an experimental model.   Arch. Environ. Health, May/June **1979**,
p. 168-172.

Sós, J.:   An investigation into the nutritional factors of experimental
cardiopathy.   Pages 161-180 in Electrolytes and Cardiovascular Disease, Volume 1, ed. by Eors Bajusz (S. Karger, Basel/New
York **1965**).   [Although Sós describes the rat diet as having "an
abundant amount of fat and cholesterol," it doesn't calculate
out to be so.   Fat figures out to be 21% of calories in both
control and cardiopathic diets.   The control diet was low
cholesterol.   The cardiopathic diet was 1% by weight, which is
only a fifth of that used by most other experimenters.]

Speich, Michelle, et al: Concentrations of magnesium, calcium,
potassium, and sodium in human heart muscle after myocardial
infarction.   Clin. Chem. 26(12): 1662-1665 (Nov **1980**)

Srivastava, U. S., et al: Mineral intakes of university students: magnesium content. Nutr. Reports Int'l. 18(2): 235-242 (Aug **1978**) Also see p. 313ff for calcium intakes.

Stallones, Reuel A.: The rise and fall of ischemic heart disease. Scientific American 243(5): 53-59 (Nov **1980**)

Stat. Abs.: Statistical Abstracts of the U. S. **1984.** (U. S. Dep't. of Commerce, Bureau of the Census) [See Table 201 for cheese and milk consumption.]

Szelenyi, I.: Magnesium and its significance in cardiovascular and gastro-intestinal disorders. World Review of Nutrition and Dietetics 17: 189-224 (**1973**)

Taylor, C. Bruce, and Shi-Kaung Peng: Vitamin D—its excessive use in the U. S. A. Pages 131-138 in Nutritional Elements and Clinical Biochemistry, ed. by Marge A. Brewster and Herbert K. Naito. (Plenum **1980**)

Terpstra, Anthony H. M.: The role of dietary protein in cholesterol metabolism. Wld. Rev. Nutr. Dietet. 42: 1-55 (**1983**)

Thakur, C. P., and A. N. Jha: Influence of milk, yoghurt and calcium on cholesterol-induced atherosclerosis in rabbits. Atherosclerosis 39: 211-215 (May **1981**)

Thompson, Paul D., et al: Incidence of death during jogging in Rhode Island from 1975 through 1980. JAMA 247(18): 2535-2538 (14 May **1982**)

Trowell, H. C., and D. P. Burkitt: Western Diseases: Their Emergence and Prevention. (Harvard Univ. Press **1981**)

Turlapaty, Prasad D. M. V., and Burton M. Altura: Magnesium deficiency produces spasms of coronary arteries: relationship to etiology of sudden death ischemic heart disease. Science 208: 198-200 (11 Apr **1980**)

Turpeinen, Osmo: Effect of cholesterol-lowering diet on mortality from coronary heart disease and other causes. Circ. 59: 1-7 (Jan **1979**) [Shows total fat consumption in Western countries.]

Varo, P.: Mineral element balance and coronary heart disease. Internat. J. Vit. Nutr. Res. 44: 267-273 (**1974**)

Venugopal, B., and T. D. Luckey: Metal Toxicity in Mammals, Volume 2. (Plenum **1978**) See pages 76-86 for cadmium toxicity.

Verlangieri, A. J., et al: Fruit and vegetable consumption and cardiovascular mortality. Medical Hypotheses 16(1): 7-15. (Jan **1985**)

Verrier, Richard L., and Bernard Lown: Neural influences and sudden cardiac death. Adv. Cardiol. 25: 155-168 (**1978**)

Vivier, C.: A theory on coronary spasm. (Letter) So. Afr. Med. J., 24 Feb **1979**, p. 275

Wacker, Warren E. C.: Magnesium and Man. (Harvard University Press **1980**)

Wadsworth, George: The Diet and Health of Isolated Populations. (CRC Press **1984**)

Walker, Mabel A., and Louise Page: Nutritive content of college meals. J. Am. Dietet. Assoc. 70: 260-266 (March **1977**)

Watson, George: Nutrition and Your Mind: The Psychochemical Response. (Harper and Row **1972**)

ABOUT THE AUTHOR

David A. Keiper graduated from Cornell University in 1953 with a degree in Engineering Physics, a five-year program with emphasis on mathematics, physics and engineering. He later had four years of graduate studies toward the Ph.D. at the University of Pennsylvania. Studies were mainly in the fields of zoology, physiology, molecular biology, biophysics and biochemistry.

His career as a research scientist, divided between applied physics and medical biophysics, included employment at The Franklin Institute Laboratories for Research and Development, Philco Corporation, and Carrier Corporation.

Since 1963, he has been involved in independent research and consulting. He has also taught college physics. He is best known and honored for having invented and developed the world's first hydrofoil sailing yacht, a 32-footer that he tested and cruised 20,000 miles around the Pacific.

Much of his research and writings have been published, both technical research papers and popular articles.

His attention began turning toward the field of nutrition about 1973. Since 1977, his particular interest has been on the relationships between nutrition and heart disease.

Index

Accidents, 4, 11, 79-80
Acne, 95
Adrenaline, 34, 70, 71
Agriculture, 21, 99-100, 137, 151
Alcohol, 11, 55-56, 66, 72-74, 79, 97, 104, 106, 109
Allergy, 17, 21, 53, 79, 83, 84, 85, 91, 92, 94, 97, 101, 111, 121
Aluminum (Al), 100, 102-103, 157, 158, 161
Amino acids, 31-32
Anemia, 92, 129, 136
Angina pectoris (chest pains), 50, 130, 133
Antibiotic side effects, 126, 131, 133
Arginine, 94, 152
Arrhythmia, 50, 52, 75, 76, 133, 136, 149
Arsenic (As), 31, 103, 138, 161
Asbestos, 67, 70
Ascorbate/ascorbic acid (see Vitamin C)
Atherosclerosis, 25, 46-48, 50-52, 56, 60, 62, 124-125, 130, 145-152
Attractiveness, sexual, 87-88, 90-95

Backache, 96
Beer, 109
Beta-blocker, 12, 96
BHT (butylated hydroxytoluene), 94, 99
Bioflavonoids, 83, 93, 94, 121, 131
Biotin, 29, 36, 125-126
Body-odor, excessive, 92, 133

Bruising, easy, 131
Bruxism, 57

Cadmium (Cd), 86, 97, 100, 103, 161
Calcium (Ca), 25, 27, 30, 38-45, 47, 50, 55-58, 61, 70, 73, 75, 85, 91, 102, 108, 132, 158-159
Calories, 28, 65-66
Cancer, 4, 23, 35, 66, 67, 68-69, 70, 100, 105, 131
Carbohydrate loading, 75
Carbohydrates, 21, 27, 28, 32-33, 37, 44, 53, 65, 75, 84, 112
Cardiovascular disease (see Coronary heart disease or Heart disease)
Carnitine (L-carnitine), 30, 36, 75
Casein, 55, 152
Cheese, 10, 21, 41, 43, 53-55, 57-58, 107, 113, 134
Chelate, 29, 134
Childhood disorders, 86, 102
Cholesterol, 4, 34, 46-48, 59-62, 147-152
Choline, 29, 34, 61, 83, 126
Chromium (Cr), 30, 33, 36, 55, 61, 83, 84, 85, 137-138, 160
Cobalt (Co), 24, 30, 36, 109
Cocaine, 32, 78
Coffee, 76, 78, 137
Congestive heart failure, 51, 130, 133
Copper (Cu), 30, 36, 61, 80, 82, 83, 89, 90, 91, 92, 96, 100, 127-128, 135-136, 159

178

Coronary artery spasms, 50, 52, 78, 148
Coronary heart disease/CHD (see also Heart attacks, Heart disease, or Sudden cardiac death), 3-19, 25, 36-52, 54-56, 59-61, 63-65, 68-70, 72, 73, 74-75, 78, 88, 97, 145-152
as failure of maintenance and self-repair mechanisms, 25, 52
conceptual framework, need for a new one, 13-14, 65, 145-152
conventional approaches to, 15, 18-19, 61, 65
importance of mineral ratios in, 39-45, 47-52, 56, 148-150
multiple causes of, 50-52, 145-146
nutritional therapy for, 14-15, 60-61, 124-125, 130, 150
prevention, 15-19
primitive societies, absence in, 5, 8-9, 39, 42, 63, 64
rise and fall of, 8, 38, 54, 150
strokes, relation to, 42, 43-45
toward a unified hypothesis, 145-152
Coronary thrombosis/clot in coronary artery, 52, 130, 148-149
Cruciferous vegetables, 110

Dagestan 9
Depression, 32, 82, 83, 133
Diets
changes over time, 37-39, 63
high-protein, 21, 75, 84, 92, 112
modern civilized, 8, 10
primitive, 20, 75
low-fat/Pritikin, 60, 66, 112-113, 131
vegetarian, 9, 60, 107
Western countries, differences among, 39-45
weight-loss, 76, 112-113
whole-food movements, 39, 105
Double-blind experiments, 61, 82, 116
Drinking (see Alcohol)
Drugs, 76-78, 79
anti-nutrient effects, 77, 133

Drugs, kicking a habit, 77-78
Drug side effects, 28, 61, 77, 83, 85, 133

Eggs, 8, 32, 46, 57, 61, 62, 106, 110, 112
Eicosapentaenoic acid/EPA (also Omega-3 oil), 34, 86, 108, 125, 131, 143, 149
Electrolyte
defined, 30
derangement, 48, 51, 52, 150
minerals (see Sodium, Potassium, Magnesium, and Calcium)
Emphysema, 68
Enzymes, 28, 31, 114
Essential fatty acids, 29, 34, 61, 93, 131
Essential nutrients, 26-34
Evolution, 20
Exercise, 4, 42, 49-50, 51, 65, 74-76, 129

Fat, dietary, 5, 10, 27, 37, 38, 43, 63-66, 106, 109
Fat-cholesterol hypothesis, 8, 65, 147-149
Fatigue, 18, 92
Fertility, 94-95
Fiber, 37, 49, 50, 61, 66, 91, 93, 111-112
Fingernails, white spots on, 83, 89, 112, 124, 136, 160
Flame-out, definition of, 3-4
Flatulence, 91, 111
Fluorine, 30, 91, 138
Food refinement (see Refinement of food)
Folic acid, 29, 36, 73, 85, 89, 92, 94, 95, 96, 126, 127, 136
Four Food Groups, 56, 106-107
Free radicals, 98-99, 129

Glucose tolerance factor (GTF-chromium), 30, 83-84, 137, 160
Glutamine, 32, 74
Glycemic index, 84
Gout, 96, 131, 136

Hair loss, 92
Hair mineral analysis, 85, 115, 155-161

Hard water, 24, 49
Heart, nutrients required by, 36
Heart attack, 3-4, 8, 9, 14-15, 18,
    47, 54, 61, 72-75, 78, 80
Heart disease, 8, 51, 97, 130, 133
    (see Coronary heart disease)
Heart rhythm (see Arrhythmia)
Hemorrhoids, 87, 93, 130
Heroin, 77-78
Herpes, 94
High blood pressure
    (see Hypertension)
High-density lipoprotein (HDL),
    34, 65, 75
High-protein diet (see Diets)
Histamine, 89-90
Homogenization of milk, 55
Hunza, 105
Hypertension (high blood
    pressure), 44, 69, 96-97, 130,
    134, 135
Hypoglycemia, 33, 79, 83-85

Immune system, 72, 93-94, 131
Individual differences, 2, 22, 36,
    61, 82, 97, 99, 114-119
Infertility, 94-95
Inositol, 29, 34, 61, 83, 127
Insecticides, 97, 99-100, 125
Insomnia, 32, 83, 125, 127, 133
Interactions
    at the molecular level, 27-28
    between bad habits and
        nutrients, 5, 10, 67-80
    between nutrients, 31, 121-139
    between toxic metals and
        nutrients, 25, 101-103
Intermittent claudication, 130
Iodine (I), 24, 30, 92, 138
Ions
    air, 24, 80
    in solution (electrolytes), 27, 30
Irish-brothers experiment, 49-50
Iron (Fe), 30, 36, 73, 82-83, 92
    102, 136-137, 159
Ischemic heart disease (see
    Coronary heart disease)

Kidney failure, 57, 97, 133
Kidney stones, 128

Lactose (milk sugar), 55, 102, 152
Lactose intolerance, 53, 54

Lead (Pb), 25, 52, 55, 79, 83, 86,
    93, 97, 102, 156, 158, 160
Lecithin, 34, 61, 70, 127
Life expectancy
    male, middle-aged, 22
    male/female difference, 1,
        11-13, 141
Linseed/flaxseed oil
    (see Eicosapentaenoic acid)
Lipids, 33-34
Lysine, 32, 94, 152
Low blood sugar
    (see Hypoglycemia)
Low-density lipoprotein (LDL),
    34, 65

Magnesium
    and arrhythmia, 50, 148
    and atherosclerosis, 50, 51
    and blood clotting, 50, 148-149
    and cholesterol, 46, 62, 147-148
    and coronary artery spasms,
        50, 148
    and dietary drift, 37, 38
    and electrolyte derangement,
        51, 52
    and exercise, 51, 74
    and experimental rat CHD, 47,
        48, 147-148
    and hard water, 49
    and sudden cardiac death, 49, 52
    and toxic metals Pb and Al,
        25, 102
    and unified hypothesis of CHD,
        147-149
    and ventricular fibrillation,
        50, 148
    and vicious circle, 51, 71-72
    as cofactor in energy
        production, 50
    as electrolyte, 30
    as regulator of Calcium, Sodium
        and Potassium, 50, 56
    benefits of supplements, 57, 61,
        70, 83, 91, 96, 97, 102,
        112, 125, 148-150
    body regulation of, 48
    deficiency in Western diets, 36,
        56, 74
    effects on brain or mental func-
        tioning, 83, 96, 125, 133
    food sources, 44, 49, 57, 134
    function in "ion" pump, 50

Magnesium [continued]
    hair levels, interpretation of,
        158-159
    importance of Ca/Mg in CHD,
        39-45, 47, 148-150
    Irish brothers study, 49-50
    loss by drinking alcohol, 48, 73
    loss in high-protein diet, 112
    loss by stress, 48, 51, 71-72
    loss by eating sugar, 48
    selective depletion in heart
        muscle cells, 50, 133
    supplements, 57, 133-134
    symptoms of deficiency,
        125, 133
    tests for cellular levels, 133
Male, causes of death, 11, 13
Manganese (Mn), 30, 36, 61, 85, 92,
    132-133, 137, 160
Masai, 5, 39-42, 49, 63
Meat, 8, 9, 20-21, 32, 39, 44,
    79, 107, 110, 130
Mental problems, 81-86, 103, 119,
    125, 161
Memory, nutrients for a failing
    memory, 83, 124, 126, 133
Mercury (Hg), 103, 161
Metabolism, defined, 28
Methionine, 46, 85, 102, 130
Milk, 10, 32, 38, 39, 44, 46, 48,
    53-58, 69, 79, 104, 106, 107
    108, 130, 137
Mineral nutrients, 24-25, 28-31,
    39-45, 132-139
Minerals, toxic, 25, 30, 101-103,
    160-161
Minoxidil, 92
Mitochondria, 35
Myocardial infarction
    (see Heart attack)

Niacin/niacinamide/nicotinic acid,
    29, 61, 73, 77, 85-86, 90, 124
Nickel (Ni), 31, 61, 92, 138
Nutrient density, 33, 63, 107
Nutrient dependencies, 120,
    124, 125
Nutrient imbalances, 30, 32, 36,
    47-48, 52, 67, 82-83, 139
Nutritional needs, male/female
    differences, 2, 45, 56, 65,
    79, 89, 92, 93, 96, 136
Nutritional practitioners, 115-118

Nutritional therapy, 14-15, 17-18,
    60-61, 114-118

Obesity, 76, 90, 97
Oils, 33-34
Olympics, ancient, 21
Omega-3 oil
    (see Eicosapentaenoic acid)
Optimum health, defined, 1

Pangamic acid, 30, 36, 61, 94, 131
Pantothenic acid, 29, 82, 92, 124
Paraaminobenzoic acid (PABA),
    29, 92, 127
Paunch, 90
Pesticides, 97, 99-100, 125
Phosphorus (P), 27, 30, 55, 91, 112,
    127, 132-133
Phytates, 110
Platelet clumping/blood platelet
    aggregation, 51, 70, 148-149
Polyunsaturated oils, 33-34, 64,
    65, 94, 96, 130, 131
Potassium (K), 30, 36, 50, 97, 135,
    158-159
Prevention of disease, 15-19
Primitive diet (see Diets)
Pritikin (see Diets, low-fat)
Prostaglandins, 19, 145
Prostate gland, 93, 136
Protective factors, dietary, 10, 44,
    55, 63, 110
Protective mechanisms, 24-26, 98
Protein, 27, 28, 31-32, 37, 94, 95,
    107, 110, 112
Pulse test for allergy, 53, 111

Rancidity of oils, 34, 64, 98,
    108, 129
RDA (see U. S. RDA)
Reducing diets
    (see Diets, weight loss)
Refinement of food, loss of
    nutrients from, 22, 32-33,
    44, 109, 129, 135, 137
    138-139

Salt (see Sodium)
Scientific method, 5-7, 13-14, 23,
    29, 39, 43, 46, 67-68, 82
Selenium (Se), 24, 30, 36, 69, 75,
    91, 99, 102, 103, 138, 156, 160
Self-therapy, 115, 118, 153-161

Sex and nutrition, 87-97
Side-effects of drugs (see Drugs)
Silicon (Si), 31, 36, 61, 90-91, 138
Sleep disorders (see Insomnia)
Smoking, 4, 11, 67, 68-70, 150
Snoring, 92
Sodium/Na (salt), 10, 30, 36, 42,
    43, 45, 47, 50, 56-57, 97,
    134, 135, 158-159
Soft drinks, 57, 133
Soils, mineral lack in, 23-24,
    69, 74, 137
Steroids, 34, 75-76
Stress, 5, 48, 51, 59-60, 71-72, 73,
    96, 132
Strokes 42, 43-45, 69, 73, 97, 134
Stuttering, 96
Sudden cardiac death (see also
        Coronary heart disease)
    and water hardness, 49
    among runners, 74-75
    rat experiments, 47-48
    scurvy, 39
    warning signs, 2, 18, 52, 102,
        133, 149, 159
Sugar (simple carbohydrate), 10,
    21, 26, 32-33, 37, 44, 48, 79,
    84, 104, 105, 106, 109
Sulfur (S), 24, 30, 46
Supplements, vitamin/mineral,
    proper use of, 119-139
    recommendations, 143-144
Synergism, 9, 67, 69

Tastes, innate, 17, 26, 63,
    66, 104-105
Teeth, 8, 91
Testosterone, 12, 34, 45, 88, 145
Thiamine (see Vitamin B-1)
Thyroid function, 92, 110, 130, 145
Toxic metals, 25, 30, 101-103,
    160-161
Trace elements, 29, 30, 31, 36-38,
    44, 45, 49, 70 (also see
        specific elements)
Tryglycerides, 33, 34
Tryptophan, 32, 83
Tyrosine, 32, 78

Ulcers, 54, 136
U. S. RDA (Recommended Dietary
    Allowance), 40, 41, 45, 101
Vanadium (V), 31, 61, 138

Varicose veins, 93, 130
Vegetable oils, 33
Vegetarian diet (see Diets)
Ventricular fibrillation,
    50-51, 148
Vicious circle, 35, 51, 72
Violence, 4, 11, 78-79
Vitamin A, 36, 61, 70, 73, 93, 94,
    95, 97, 99, 101, 122-123
Vitamin B-1 (thiamine), 36, 73, 91,
    96, 123
Vitamin B-2 (riboflavin), 123
Vitamin B-3 (see Niacin)
Vitamin B-5
    (see Pantothenic acid)
Vitamin B-6 (pyridoxine), 36, 38,
    49, 61, 70, 73, 83, 85, 90, 91,
    93, 94, 95, 124-125, 136
Vitamin B-12 (cobalamin), 73, 85,
    92, 94, 95, 125
Vitamin B-15 (see Pangamic acid)
Vitamin C, 16, 36. 38, 47, 61, 65,
    66, 70, 72, 73, 75, 77, 82, 83,
    85, 86, 90, 91, 93, 94, 95, 96,
    97, 99, 101, 102, 127-128
Vitamin D, 34, 36, 38, 47, 64, 128
Vitamin E, 34, 36-38, 49, 65, 66,
    70, 73, 75, 83, 93, 94, 95, 99,
    101, 102, 128-131
Vitamin F
    (see Essential fatty acids)
Vitamin K, 131
Vitamin P (see Bioflavonoids)
Vitamins, B-complex, 29-30, 70,
    75, 82, 83, 92, 123
Vitamins, list of, 29-30

Water, drinking, 98, 99, 100
Water hardness, 49
Whole-food movements, 39, 105
World Health Organization
    (WHO), recommendations of,
    40, 41, 45, 56

Xanthine oxidase, 55, 146

Yogurt, 10, 21, 39-44, 53-55,
    57-58, 61, 106, 126, 134,
    151, 152

Zinc (Zn), 24, 30, 36, 73, 75, 80,
    82, 83, 85, 89, 92, 93, 94, 95,
    97, 102, 135-136, 156, 160